CHOOSE THE SEX

CHOOSE THE SEX OF YOUR BABY

The Natural Way

—————

Hazel Chesterman-Phillips

BLOOMSBURY

First published in 1997 by Bloomsbury Publishing plc
2 Soho Square
London, W1V 6HB

Copyright © 1997 by Hazel Chesterman-Phillips

The moral right of the author has been asserted

A copy of the CIP entry for this book is available from the British Library

ISBN 0 7475 3057 2

10 9 8 7 6 5 4 3 2 1

Jacket design by Fielding Rowinski
Designed by AB3
Illustrations by Chartwell Illustrators
Typeset by Hewer Text Composition Services, Edinburgh
Printed in Great Britain by Clays Ltd, St Ives plc

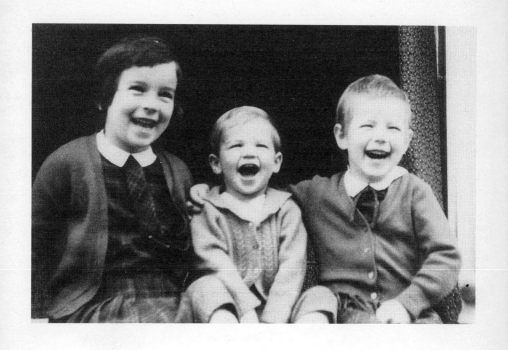

Sheena   Dick   Penny
To our mixed family

And to my co-operative husband who made it possible

ACKNOWLEDGEMENTS

I am most grateful to my father, Sir Clement Chesterman, OBE, MD, FRCP, for his constant interest and encouragement. Before he died, he said to me, 'You may well have something there, my dear. Pursue it.' And so I have.

Thanks also to my family:

To my girls for giving me the idea in the first place and for forgiving me for calling them 'mistakes'.

To my boy for upholding the theory and being conceived on the day of ovulation.

To my obliging husband for doing everything just right. And then for providing me with *le mot juste* whenever I got stuck in the writing of this book.

Many thanks to all the doctors who spared time to send me information and advice. Their comments were invaluable.

And to the libraries of Barnet and St Marylebone and the Royal College of Physicians who unfailingly supplied me with books and articles from Britain and abroad.

I am indebted to Professor Robert Winston for much of the physiological information contained in Chapter 1.

Finally, my heartfelt gratitude to all the families who put my theory to the test and who had the guts to write and tell me in such eloquent letters, whether successful or sad, about their experiences in choosing the sex of their baby.

CONTENTS

INTRODUCTION

This book is the account of my experience as a woman who very much wanted a mixed family, thought a great deal about it and found a natural way which proved successful. Having already had two daughters, I read all I could find in 1960 on the subject of sex determination, and pondered on it, trying to discover a natural law for sex selection. I worked out a formula and used it to get our son, born in 1963.

Over the next ten years, I passed the method on to forty friends and relations of child-bearing age who were keen to choose the sex of their next child and, in this forty, there was 100 per cent success in choosing the sex of the baby.

The journalist Tessa Hilton wrote the theory up for *Mother & Baby* magazine, and through this journal's wide circulation, the method travelled to many countries from Britain to New Zealand. Immense feedback came from women all over the world who had tried the method. Their experiences gave me the fascinating raw material for this book. The theory that had worked for me and my husband was also working for other couples too!

In 1976, there was an article in a British magazine by the American gynaecologist, Dr Landrum B. Shettles, who was well known in the United States for his research into sex selection. He put forward in medical jargon ideas very similar to those contained in my theory of sex selection. I was gratified to see how closely we agreed. And I was glad that my son was already a strapping lad of thirteen years, which nicely provided proof that my ideas had come from an independent source years before Dr Shettles' book appeared in America in 1970.

From 1978–88, I checked on my hunches while studying for a degree at the Open University in science and philosophy. I further found that my ideas were shared by a number of doctors in various countries with whom I then began to correspond. This book sets out the rules for anyone to try. I put them forward here as a guiding light for women who are floundering, as I was, in the frustration of not knowing how to produce a child of the sex they desire. They cannot afford to wait for scientific proof. Perhaps they would like to try this natural method which worked for me three times and for so many others.

If women can quickly produce their desired family of chosen sex, perhaps it will act as an incentive to stop bearing more children. Many women, quite naturally, carry on trying for children if so far they have had children of only one sex. Being able to choose the sex of your child can mean smaller families. I believe this could help to check one of the most pressing crises of our time – the population explosion of the world.

CHAPTER 1

THE EGG

The Female Reproductive System – from egg (ovum) to ovulation

---

For some people there appears to be no problem in choosing the sex of their baby. Careful Kate read the rules for a girl in a friend's book. She spent six months observing her menstrual cycle and then went on holiday with her husband and two sons. Her husband adjusted his sperm count, she followed the timing rules exactly – and fell pregnant. Nine months later, their daughter was born, to the family's delight and satisfaction.

For the more reckless, success takes longer. Second-wife Tracy wrote:

We were hoping for a boy but I'm afraid we were not strict enough with ourselves. We romantically followed our feelings and made love too often and too soon. We got a girl – my husband's fifth! The second time we tried I and my husband stuck sternly to all the rules for a boy. I personally supervised the ice-cold swim before dinner while we were on holiday in Lanzarote. Thirty-six weeks later, I delivered a bouncing seven and a half pound BOY! Little David is a dream come true. My husband is still suffering from shock!

What are these rules that are so strict and uncompromising? If we conform fully, the result is what we expect; if we deviate from the rule, the result changes accordingly. Nature's rules are fixed but we humans sometimes make a mistake. How can we discover these rules so that we can carry them out perfectly and get the child of our choice every time?

Let us investigate the very beginnings of human life and learn a little of how nature works. The egg, the female sex cell (gamete), is a good place to start as all higher animal life begins there. This small, smooth sphere holds the template of life from which we all originate. And it also promotes life for the future. When the egg is fertilized in the woman's body, it immediately reduplicates itself and produces more eggs for the next generation. The egg first makes sure of its descendants. Such is the cunning stratagem of a natural system that exists by the rule of the survival of the fittest.

The process which produces ova begins when the human female embryo is less than two millimetres long – about twenty-one days after fertilization. Egg-producing cells are called primordial germ cells. About one hundred of these quickly migrate to the tissues in the foetus which will become the ovaries. Here they multiply continuously.

After five months in the womb, a baby girl has around 7 million eggs in her ovaries. Most of these die before she is born when there will be only 2 million left. At puberty, half a million remain. Of these, only a few, 400–500 will actually be ovulated, one per month, in an adult woman's menstrual cycle.

A diploid cell is one which carries the full number of chromosomes characteristic of the species. But by the time of ovulation when the egg emerges from the ovary on its way to be fertilized, it will be a haploid cell, one containing only half the normal 46 gene-carrying chromosomes that all other adult cells have. A process called meiosis (*see page 16, Chapter 3*) will have reduced the number to 23. The other 23 will be supplied by the sperm which fertilizes the egg. These two sets of genes determine the genetic make-up of the baby and decide its unique characteristics.

Human eggs are stored in the ovaries. Some of them may remain here for forty years, the duration of a woman's fertility. This fact may explain why older women who shed eggs towards the end of their reproductive life are at greater risk of conceiving a genetically damaged child, springing from a somewhat stale egg perhaps.

The immature eggs lie quiescent all through a girl's childhood until puberty when some of them respond to hormone messages sent by the pituitary gland, the master of all hormone-producing endocrine glands. The pituitary gland lies at the base of the brain, behind the eye-sockets and in front of the hypothalamus, a control centre which is thought to influence the pituitary to produce these hormones: Follicle Stimulating Hormone (FSH) and Luteinizing Hormone (LH).

FSH stimulates eggs to become mature inside a small blister-like structure inside the ovary called a Graafian follicle (so-named after the Dutch anatomist, Regnier de Graaf, who discovered it in 1670). This organ is filled with fluid and the egg usually grows to one side of the follicle – anticipating the fertilized egg later implanting itself on the side of the womb.

At this time, the egg needs a lot of energy as it is highly active while it is maturing in the run up to ovulation. To obtain this energy it needs to absorb more of the oxygen which diffuses over its surface area from the atmosphere outside. The egg itself receives no help from its own structure to provide the energy it needs, as it is a virtually perfect sphere of smooth shape which provides the smallest surface area possible for its size. But 7 million granulosa helper cells surround each egg and line each follicle. The total surface area of these cells greatly increases the amount of energy available to the egg by absorption. Thus the tiny egg cell is serviced by millions of granulosa cells as assiduously as worker bees serve their Queen.

The granulosa cells are also instrumental in sending chemical messages to the brain to trigger ovulation. Professor Robert Winston of London's Hammersmith Hospital describes what is known as a 'Feedback Mechanism' like this:

> As FSH stimulates the follicle to grow, the granulosa cells (which produce oestrogen) increase in number and activity. As the granulosa cells increase, so does the manufacture of oestrogen. Eventually oestrogen output is high and some of it gets into the bloodstream. This rise in oestrogen in the blood stimulates the brain, telling the hypothalamus that the follicle is now mature and ready to release a ripe egg. An immediate message is then sent from the hypothalamus to the pituitary gland. The pituitary responds by sending out a sharp pulse of LH, and approximately 36 hours after the rise of LH in the blood the follicle opens and releases the egg. Ovulation occurs.

This paragraph nicely explains the working of the fertility kits that many women use to help them determine their day of ovulation (*see page 82, Chapter 9*). The phrase to be noted is: *approximately* 36 hours *after* the rise of LH in the blood, ovulation occurs.

Yasmin was trying for a son. Because she had irregular periods, she decided to use a Clearplan Ovulation Kit to find her day of ovulation. The blue line duly appeared in the large window and intercourse took place immediately.

Nine months later, Yasmin gave birth to a second daughter.

What Yasmin failed to do when Clearplan showed the blue line, was to *wait* a bit longer for the ovulatory vaginal mucus to appear before making love in order for her to conceive a son. Medical research says 'up to 36 hours later'. But all women are different and mould the rule to their personal rhythm. The 36 hours may extend to 48 hours in some cases. The only safe thing to do after the Ovulation Kit shows the required colour, is to look out for the slippery vaginal mucus that denotes ovulation (*see page 77, Chapter 9*). This mucus is the most accurate indication of ovulation. *Then* is the time to make love for a son.

Sadly, Yasmin made love too soon, before she had ovulated. Hence she conceived a daughter – according to the precision of nature's rule. We will look into this in more detail in Chapter 9.

We return now to the egg. After ovulation, the egg will probably find its way into one of the Fallopian tubes (so named after their Italian discoverer in 1562, Gabriele Fallopius). As it travels along towards the womb in this tube, it may become fertilized by a sperm.

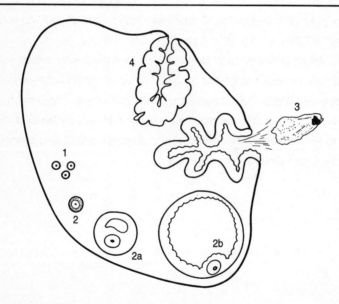

The development of a follicle containing the egg. (1) Immature eggs. (2, 2a & 2b) Maturing Graafian follicle and egg. (3) Rupture of follicle with release of egg surrounded by granulosa cells (ovulation). (4) Corpus luteum about 4–5 days after ovulation.

Fig. 1: Ovulation

Meanwhile, another feedback mechanism is taking place. Stimulated by the pituitary gland's release of LH before ovulation, the granulosa cells start to manufacture a second hormone, progesterone. This hormone prepares the uterus for the implantation of the developing embryo, if fertilization has successfully occurred.

The granulosa cells also make a bright yellow pigment which stains the ruptured follicle, making it into a yellow body (corpus luteum). This structure also starts to produce progesterone which is essential for the early development of the embryo. If the corpus luteum is damaged, there may be an early miscarriage.

Thus at ovulation, the egg leaves the ovary on its way to make a new human being.

Ovulation occurs when the follicle bursts open and the egg leaves the ovary. (This event may be the cause of the sharp ovulatory pain which some women experience.) In humans, this happens usually half-way between menstrual cycles, i.e. on day 14 in a standard 28 day cycle. This gives the egg fourteen days to travel down the Fallopian tube to the womb.

But, as I have already said, the actual day of ovulation varies from woman to woman and sometimes from cycle to cycle. Every woman must discover her own ovulation day. Personally, I was lucky enough to have a regular short cycle of 24 days with ovulation occurring on Day 10. For those who find ovulation difficult to determine there are many aids to help you, and I refer to these in detail later in Chapter 9.

CHAPTER 2

THE SPERM

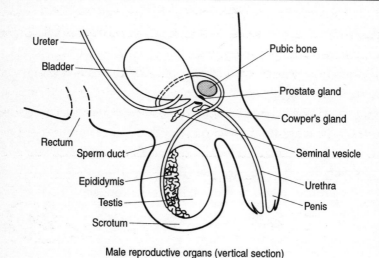

Male reproductive organs (vertical section)

Fig. 2: The Male Reproductive System

Sperm (male gametes) are made in the testes. These hang in the scrotum away from the body – which keeps them a bit below body temperature. Coolness encourages sperm production.

The testes start producing sex cells at puberty (from about 13 years of age onwards) when they respond to hormone messages sent by the pituitary gland. Follicle Stimulating Hormone (FSH) stimulates male sperm gametes at puberty just as it stimulates female egg gametes (*see page 4, Chapter 1*).

The sperm are transported by rhythmic contractions along the tubes of the epididymis where they remain for 2–3 weeks and gain the ability to move (motility). Under their own power they swim out into the vas deferens which leads down the penis to the exterior, or into the female tract during intercourse. As they go, secretions are added to the sperm from the seminal vesicle and the prostate gland. These secretions do two things:

1 They supply food to provide energy for the sperms' motility.

2 They counteract the acidity inside the female tract.

Meanwhile, mucus secreted by the Cowper's glands blocks off the urethra.

Just as the egg is the largest cell in the body, the sperm is the smallest. Another haploid cell (*see page 4, Chapter 1*), it is like a tiny missile made up of three major parts:

1 The *head*, which contains the sperm's genetic information lying on 23 chromosomes – half the number needed for full diploid cells. The head is surrounded by a cap, an aerosome, which is not removed until just before fertilization; rather like the arming of a warhead.

2 The *mid-piece*, a complex structure carrying fuel and computer systems to control movement.

3 The *whiplash tail*, which propels the sperm forward. The sperm accelerates considerably as it approaches the egg.

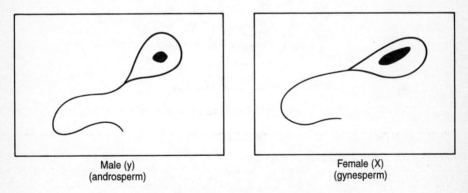

Male (y)
(androsperm)

Female (X)
(gynesperm)

Fig. 3: The Two Kinds of Sperm

The female-bearing, oval-headed X gynesperm are larger, slower and live longer. They have greater staying power against the hazards of the vaginal environment and some can survive for 5–6 days in the woman's body after they have been ejaculated.

The male-bearing, round-headed androsperm are smaller, but have longer tails which makes them faster and more agile. However, they do not survive for so long. Normal androsperm die off after 2 days though occasionally, in very fertile men, they live longer (*see page 59, Chapter 8*).

The woman ovulates once a menstrual month, releasing an ovum (X) (*see page 13, Chapter 3*), which has potential for female or male production, i.e. if it is fertilized, it can produce either a girl or a boy. The man's sperm, one of which may fertilize the X ovum, is made up of a mixture of X and y sperm, almost invariably fifty-fifty. It is exceedingly rare for a man not to have such a mixture.

'The number of cases in which men are able to produce only one sex is too insignificant to warrant the expense and inconvenience of tests to find out. Most doctors are not equipped to carry out such tests anyway,' says Dr Landrum Shettles, the American sex determination expert.

I stress this point because of the many letters I get from mothers of single-sex families who are convinced that their husbands do not have sperm of the other sex. Like Karen (*see page 31, Chapter 5*) they are not persuaded until they have tried the method and proved their husband is as normal as everyone else!

The sex of the baby is determined by the first sperm to fertilize the ovum.

If the man's X sperm fertilizes the ovum, a girl will be conceived.
If the man's y sperm fertilizes the ovum, a boy will be conceived.

$$X \text{ ovum} + X \text{ sperm} = 2X = a \text{ girl}$$
$$X \text{ ovum} + y \text{ sperm} = Xy = a \text{ boy}$$

Thus it is the man who genetically determines the sex of a baby. How does this happen? How does the presence of a y chromosome assign maleness to a developing foetus?

In an article in the *Guardian*, Saffron Davies wrote:

'*For six or seven weeks after fertilization, the foetus remains in a sexual limbo, waiting to see what sex it will be. The fertilized embryo has potentiality for either sex as it contains the rudiments of testicles and ovaries.*

The testes await a chemical signal from the male androsperm to kick them into action. The male y chromosome contains a tiny gene which produces a putative chemical message (arbitrarily called the 'Testis Determining Factor'). On receipt of this message, the testes produce a sudden spurt of progesterone which stimulates the production of penis and scrotum. Thus it is ensured that male sexual characteristics proceed and female development is sternly suppressed.

It occurs to me that, if we could fully understand this mechanism, we might discover another method of sex determination?

SPERM COUNT

A sperm count is the analysis of a man's sperm: of the semen and of the number, health and motility of the sperm in one ejaculate. A sample of sperm is examined under the microscope for the following qualities:

1 Semen volume: Normally, 2–5 millilitres (up to one teaspoonful) per ejaculation. If less, the man may not be producing enough seminal fluid. If more, the seminal fluid may dilute the sperm too much.
2 Sperm numbers: Should be greater than 40 million per millilitre. Below 20 million may cause a problem with fertility. Though some men are fertile with a low sperm count.
3 Sperm motility: At least 40 per cent of sperm should be active and moving.
4 Normal and defective sperm: At least 65 per cent of sperm should look normal under the microscope. A sperm count will identify any defective sperm.
5 Routine tests: check for any antibodies.

Sperm count in all men is variable and changes frequently according to different environmental conditions. Heat and sexual activity lowers it. Conversely, coolness and abstinence may raise it. Many environmental factors contribute to reduced sperm production and poor sperm quality, as you can read in Chapter 10.

CHAPTER 3

HEREDITY, GENES AND CHROMOSOMES

The main property that distinguishes living matter from all other matter, is its ability to synthesize proteins. These complex substances form the chemical basis of life.

The difference between a man and an elephant, or a man and an oak tree, or between two men, is largely the difference between the proteins they can make. This ability is what they inherit from their forbears and this is what they transmit to their offspring through their genes (see below).

Coiled up in the nucleus of every living cell is a nucleic acid called DNA (Deoxyribonucleic acid), which governs the manufacture of proteins. One length of DNA is a gene and this makes a specific protein which produces a unique characteristic of that body. A second nucleic acid, RNA (Ribonucleic acid), has the ability to replicate DNA which it then passes to the substance of the cell. Thus RNA acts as a mould and messenger for DNA in the synthesis of protein. The body contains thousands of different kinds of protein, each determined by the DNA in the cell nucleus.

The fertilized ovum (zygote) contains in its DNA all the genetic information for the cells of its future adult body. Every cell of that body, whether in a hair or a toenail, will carry a replica of the same DNA as is in the zygote. For identification purposes, DNA is a fingerprint *par excellence*!

Before a cell divides, the genes are organized into paired structures on a rod-like particle called a chromosome. Chromosomes can be seen, under a microscope, in the nucleus of a cell during cell division. After separation they disappear; they are not seen in a resting cell (see Peter Wyngate, p. 103, Medical Dictionary, Penguin, 1978).

In an organism, chromosomes are in homologous pairs, that is to say there are in the nucleus two similar chromosomes, one inherited from each parent. These have the same DNA and carry genes determining the same proteins (and hence characteristic features) which may be inherited from either parent. Chromosomes are collections of a large number of genes, each gene determining one element in the hereditary make-up of the body.

Each chromosome in a homologous pair carries information for the same characteristics, and these genes are in the same position on both parental chromosomes.

The nucleus of a resting cell contains a jumble of genes. When the cell is about to divide, this material is arranged as a set of X- or V-shaped chromosomes.

There are 23 pairs of chromosomes in the human set. The members of a pair are similar except for the pair of sex chromosomes in the male. In the female, this twenty-third pair consists of two large X chromosomes (XX); in the male, one large X and one small y chromosome(Xy). Hence we respectively call the female-bearing gynesperm X, and the male-bearing androsperm y.

CELL DIVISION AND GROWTH IN ORDINARY CELLS – MITOSIS

The second major property of the living cell lies in its ability to grow. Growth takes place through the simple process of duplication and division. Each cell grows to an optimum size, replicates its chromosomes and then divides into two exact copies of its parent cell.

As soon as a woman's egg is fertilized, it begins to grow at a rapid rate of cell division. The chromosomes play a major part in this process which is called mitosis. Mitosis is the manner of duplication and division in the cell as it grows. Consider for example *one* chromosome in mitosis.

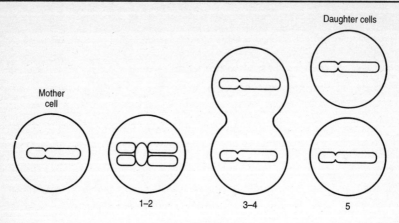

Fig. 4: Mitosis

1 The genes replicate themselves and line up in identical pairs on the chromosome.

2 The chromosome lies down the spindle, a slender structure formed in the cell during division.

3 The chromosome splits down the middle into two identical chromatids.

4 The chromatids are drawn away from each other to opposite sides of the cell.

5 The cell divides into two daughter cells identical with their mother cell, and with each other.

In an adult cell, this process occurs simultaneously in all 46 chromosomes.

CELL DIVISION IN SEX CELLS – MEIOSIS

The mitotic method of identical reproduction of the mother cell obviously will not do in the production of sex cells, because this must involve the combination of genetic material from *both* parents.

Animals that reproduce sexually have testes and ovaries. In these organs the special reproductive egg and sperm cells (gametes) produced by each parent respectively are manufactured. They fuse in fertilization to form a zygote which has a single nucleus containing the genetic material from both parents. The zygote then begins to divide mitotically and to grow into a new individual.

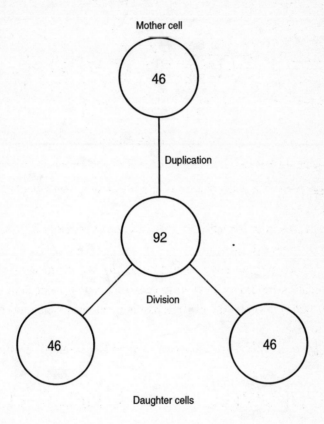

Fig. 5: Duplication and Division of Chromosomes in Mitosis

(Stylized example of a pair of homologous sex chromosomes from a diploid cell in a gonad: (ovary or testis).

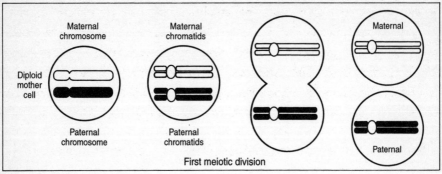

First meiotic division

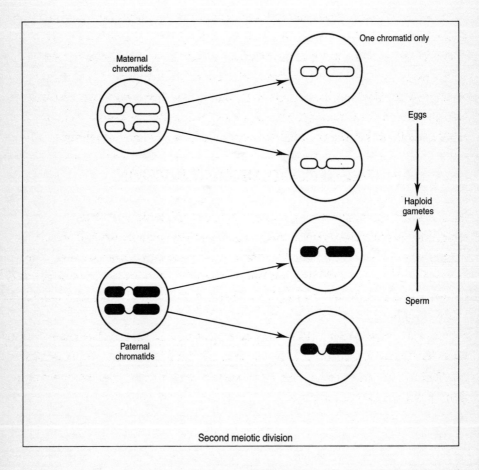

Second meiotic division

Fig. 6: Meiosis

Haploid gametes cannot be reproduced by mitosis because these daughter cells must carry only half the diploid number of chromosomes of the adult. As we saw in Chapter 1, adult cells have 46 chromosomes. Eggs and sperm must have only 23 so that when they fuse in fertilization the resulting zygote will have the normal 46 chromosomes. Meiosis is a specialized form of mitosis that reduces the number of chromosomes in the daughter cells by half.

Meiosis occurs in an elegantly simple manner, by carrying the division process one stage further in a second meiotic division.

MEIOSIS

1 The chromosomes replicate themselves into two identical chromatids.
2 The double chromatids lie down the spindle.
3 The double chromatids are drawn away from each other to opposite sides of the cell (just like the single chromatids in mitosis).
4 The cell divides into two identical daughter cells, each with two chromatids from one of the original pair of chromosomes in the gamete.

This completes the first meiotic division. It is followed immediately by:

THE SECOND MEIOTIC DIVISION

Each daughter cell, containing two chromatids from only one of the original chromosomes, divides again in mitotic division forming four haploid sex cells (egg or sperm) each with a single chromatid from only one chromosome of the original pair. These haploid granddaughter cells are 23-chromosome gametes which need to fuse with a partner to become a fertilized embryo with 46 chromosomes.

The diagram on page 18 shows how cell division in mitosis is taken a step further in meiosis reducing 46 chromosomes in a diploid cell in ovary or testis to 23 chromosomes in a haploid gamete cell. Thus heredity is passed down by both parents in equal amounts.

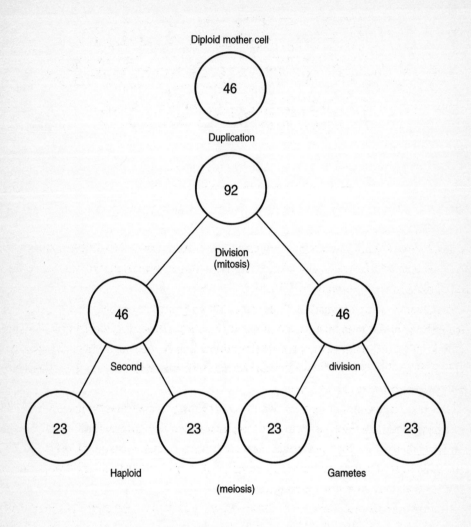

Fig. 7: **Further Reduction Through Cell Division**

CHAPTER 4

INTERCOURSE, CONCEPTION AND PREGNANCY

During sexual intercourse, between 100 million and 300 million sperm are ejaculated into the vagina. The normal volume of semen in one ejaculate is 1–8 millilitres (1 teaspoon = 5 ml).

Each sperm is genetically unique, carrying a distinctive set of genes derived from those of the man, just as each egg carries unique genetic material from the woman. Depending on which sperm first hits which egg, the resulting baby will exhibit individual characteristics from both parents according to the genes which the gametes carried.

Such a large number of sperm may seem unnecessary since only one will eventually fertilize the egg, but many sperm are needed because of the perilous journey they must face in the woman's body. Many sperm perish before they ever get into the vagina. They simply fall out in a very natural way. Couples should not worry too much about this.

Those that do make it are immediately faced with a hostile environment in the vaginal mucus which is, for the most part, thick and sticky and acid. Many sperm take a wrong turning, lose their way or die of exhaustion. Acidity is nature's way of protecting against infection and bacteria which might damage the reproductive organs. But it also rebuffs the very sperm which are crucial for the survival of the species. This seems a bit strange until one realizes that this obstacle ensures that only the strongest sperms get through. (We shall see later that these facts have a bearing on the method of sex selection described in this book.)

About 5 per cent of the sperm survive to get to the neck of the womb (cervix). Here the mucus is thin and alkaline and friendly to the sperm. When the latter come into contact with this mucus, a mysterious process called capacitation takes place in which the sperm cap (aerosome) is removed. Only when this has happened is the sperm capable of penetrating the ovum, which is waiting suitably emplaced in the Fallopian tube.

Thus within 5–10 minutes of ejaculation, the egg may be fertilized by one of the sperm that has survived this incredible journey.

Conception takes place in the Fallopian tube. This complex tunnel does much to encourage the meeting of the egg and the sperm. Its muscular contractions speed the sperms on their way to the egg in one direction while simultaneously transporting the egg in precisely the opposite direction – towards the uterus and the sperm pool. Furthermore, the Fallopian tube also acts as a filter, trapping dead or abnormal sperm so that only healthy ones arrive in the upper part, the ampulla. Here they may fertilize a suitably mature egg.

The successful sperm loses its tail on entering the egg and its head becomes a second nucleus in the cell. This pronucleus, as it is called, lies alongside the female pronucleus in the egg for a few hours before they fuse in fertilization. A mature egg allows only one single sperm to penetrate it and then immediately puts up a chemical barrier which prevents other sperm from entering. (Non-identical twins come when the woman produces two eggs and each is fertilized by a different sperm. Each of these embryos will be attached to the mother's womb by its own placenta.)

The mature egg has its chromosomes ready for division and growth and during the first 24 hours, the cell divides into two. During the next 24 hours, each of these cells divides. Thereafter, cell division occurs at intervals of about 15 hours. After three days or so, when the embryo comprises 8 cells, each cell has what is called totipotential. This means that each cell separately has the ability to develop into a human being. Thus, if the eight-celled embryo was divided into eight independent cells, each of these could grow into one of eight identical human beings. This is how identical twins occur. Sometimes the embryo divides spontaneously into two, producing two individuals with exactly the same DNA and genetic material from both parents. Such twins are always of the same sex. Fraternal twins occur when more than one egg is fertilized and both foetuses develop and grow separately. Fraternal twins are not identical and can be of different sexes.

Mothers sometimes ask me how I account for fraternal twins with my method of sex selection. I cannot.

Identical twins of the same sex presumably follow the usual rule for girls or boys. Fraternal twins of the same sex also follow the usual rules of intercourse at ovulation for boys, and intercourse before ovulation for girls. By some fluke of timing two sperm penetrate two eggs at precisely the same moment. Or sometimes at different moments.

Having already a cute little girl, Marion, my elder sister, Heather Hanbury Brown, gave birth to non-identical, fraternal twin boys who were born within ten minutes of each other but who were conceived a month apart. This was reflected in their birth weights: Robert, 7 lbs 11 oz, and Jordan, 5 lbs 1 oz. Robert was slightly overdue with long fingernails and Jordan hirsute with slight prematurity as he had had only eight months' gestation. As usual, both these boys had been conceived at ovulation. But one month apart – not usual at all! Mother and babies all flourished.

Mixed twins are a different conundrum which I cannot explain fully. If conceived after intercourse-before-ovulation, a female gynesperm must have had unusual speed; if conceived after intercourse-at-ovulation a male androsperm must have had extra staying power. Perhaps mixed twins are the result of a remarkable sperm count? I await further elucidation.

PREGNANCY

Two weeks after fertilization, the human embryo enters the uterus where it floats around for a few days, constantly dividing and multiplying although not growing in physical size at all. It remains the same size as the original egg-cell because each new cell formed is smaller than the last and packs in to the same area. The embryo is now a ball of cells round a central cavity filled with fluid. This is called a blastocyst and the woman is well and truly pregnant.

After six or seven days, the embryo starts to increase in size and implants itself into the lining of the uterus, the endometrium. Implantation is an amazing phenomenon. The embryo is an individual quite different from the mother and as such should be rejected by her as a foreign body. But the 23 maternal chromosomes must be enough to identify with the mother who accepts the embryo like a perfect transplant.

This stage of pregnancy is very precarious. Forty per cent of human embryos miscarry at this point, and many more at the time of menstruation later. If women have a slightly delayed, heavy period, this may signify the loss of an embryo. It is not known medically why this should be so. But it may be because the body has not yet caught up with the radical changes taking place, and the natural cleansing mechanism of the period continues as normal. Sometimes, tragically, the baby is being thrown out with the bath-water, as it were.

It is not surprising that mothers feel below par and even sick and ill during the first months of pregnancy. After all, we are in the process of forming the brains and nervous systems of new people. An awesome task, indeed.

After 14 days, the embryo is firmly implanted in the uterine lining and the danger of miscarriage recedes. Though mothers should still treat themselves carefully at what would have been the time of their period for the first three months. That is at 4 weeks, at 8 weeks, at 12 weeks (or whatever intervals fit your individual cycle pattern). These are times of high risk of miscarriage. If you start to bleed, go to bed immediately and lie as still as possible for a few days. I myself lost some blood at three months with both my daughters. But I went to bed for a few days and happily managed to hang on to them.

So rest up and take things as easy as possible during this time. If you have older children, get them to wait on you a bit while you are in your 'interesting condition', as the Victorians used to call it. Most young children enjoy playing nurse to mum. Make a game of it and enjoy the pregnancy together.

CHAPTER 5

WHY CHOOSE?

When she turned twelve, Jacinta's father committed suicide leaving a note saying that with five daughters approaching adulthood, he couldn't bear the shame of not being able to give them the dowries they needed. He hoped his death would raise compassion in the hearts of prospective husbands for his daughters whom he loved deeply.

Sarbjit, aged twenty-nine, had three daughters aged eight, six and five years. Pregnant again, Sarbjit waited in hope and fear until a three-month scan told her she was indeed carrying another daughter. Four weeks later, despairing at the looming prospect of future dowries, Sarbjit spun a tale of depression and financial problems when she applied for and got a termination in a Leeds hospital. After the operation, Sarbjit suffered a cardiac arrest and died.

Amina, another young mother, has been clinically depressed since the birth of her third daughter. She also spoke of suicide and dowries but cheered slightly when she heard of a new 'medication' to get a boy. But this 'medication' means sperm separation and artificial insemination at London's new Gender Clinic. This costs up to £1000. Amina is depressed again.

One suicide, one death leaving three little girls with only a single parent, and a deeply depressed mother struggling to bring up three daughters she did not really want. 'My sorrow has become my illness,' says Amina. 'I am trapped by life.'

These tragedies could have been averted but for the lack of a simple piece of knowledge which might have enabled the parents to conceive a child of the sex that could have transformed their lives.

It has been argued that the dowry system created a stable society which survived for centuries in some countries and that it would be potentially disastrous to meddle with it. But ideas change as time passes, and now it is questionable as to whether any society should be allowed to flourish when its laws can bring so much hurt to its members. Today many people, myself included, regard the dowry system as outdated and iniquitous and feel that it should be changed with all possible speed. And it *is* changing gradually, as younger generations teach us to place more importance on the personal value of girl or boy friends rather than on their financial circumstances.

However, this change is too slow to have prevented the tragic cases above. As long as their culture retain old values, individuals need to be given the chance to choose their children. Occasionally, I have been criticized for perpetuating the current state of affairs by helping women to secure the son they want so much. 'You shouldn't encourage this attitude. It is the society that is at fault and should be changed,' say my critics. But even if I agree, it is unlikely that I can change that society. And these women need their sons now. They cannot wait for a social revolution. So meanwhile, I will do all I can to relieve the suffering of such distraught women. I am reminded of the words of the song, 'If I can help somebody as I pass along, then my living will not be in vain.'

And many others desire this choice also. We have seen that in some societies the culture demands a son for various religious or socio-financial reasons. As a result, the family may bring great pressure to bear on wives to produce a son, and life can be cruelly hard for women who have only daughters.

I have two lovely daughters [wrote Kushmal] *but since my sister has had a son, no adult in my wider family takes any notice of my girls. All attention is focused on their cousin because he is a boy, and my girls get nothing. Nobody even talks to them; they are completely ignored. I am indignant and miserable. Are my daughters not worth any recognition at all?*

And this letter came from another part of England:

Please can you help me? I am so depressed and at this moment I am on the verge of suicide. My marriage is a disaster and I know there is only one thing that can save it, and that is for me to give my husband a baby son. I have a daughter but I desperately need a son. Recently my sister gave birth to her first child, a son. And now my husband shouts at me to produce one too. He argues and argues and says he wants me to leave him. Now we are sleeping in separate rooms.

But I love and need him desperately. Please help me.

Thank you,

Roshni

Nobody can be blamed for following the beliefs and customs of the tradition into which they were born. But it is salutary sometimes to stand back and consider the reasonableness of a tradition which has been passed down from the ignorance of former times. Then, it was considered the duty of a woman to provide a son for her husband. And many poor innocent women suffered when they had the bad luck to bear daughters. But nowadays we know more about the timing and sperm count factors which determine the sex of a new baby. Timing depends on the woman but sperm count is entirely the man's responsibility, and it is cruel and ignorant to hold the woman solely responsible for the sex of the baby produced.

It is ironic that a man should blame his wife for not producing a son. True, she may not have got the timing of intercourse right, but the mistake may not lie with her at all. It could be due to the man's sperm count which may have been too low when he tried to beget a son. If he leaves this wife and goes to another, he will probably beget three more girls! Exactly this happened to the Lord of a Stately Home in the English Midlands. Desperate for an heir, he flitted from wife to wife. Now he has six daughters!

Because there are so many variables in husband *and* wife which are influential in determining the sex of the baby, it is best if the couple work together as a team in choosing the sex of their child. The unchosen sex of a baby is nobody's *fault*. It is usually the sad outcome of ignorance. Both parents will probably be badly disappointed and deserve all the love and support a family can give. This is a vastly preferable course to take rather than fruitlessly resenting the innocent child and his/her unhappy mother.

Nature may be cruel and unfair in many aspects, but she is not unfair in the game of sex determination. The rules are fixed and unswerving. If we follow them precisely, we get the child of the sex we choose. Our difficulty lies in learning all the various rules for men *and* women, and obeying them accurately.

Sometimes, physical problems may necessitate the desire to choose a certain sex. Muscular dystrophy is one of the hereditary diseases which is carried by girls but which only affects boys from time to time. It is generally accepted in Britain now that women who carry such diseases should be tested in pregnancy and given the option of a termination if the foetus is affected.

Christine and Sue were both pregnant and carrying girls. They knew the sex of their babies because they had been treated by Professor Robert Winston. Both women carry the gene for muscular dystrophy. This illness has already meant a death sentence within ten years for Sue's elder six-year-old son, David, who has been crushingly diagnosed as suffering from the disease.

To prevent the recurrence of such a tragedy, Sue and Christine turned to Professor Winston for his method of In Vitro Fertilization (IVF). Here, eggs are fertilized in a glass petri dish outside the woman's body and the embryos tested to determine their sex. Then only girl embryos are replaced in the womb. Hence the mothers know, thanks to such brilliant technology, that they are carrying daughters.

But brilliant technology is expensive and often traumatic for the parents. How much better if Sue and Christine had been able, by natural conception, to choose the daughters they wanted so much.

Unfortunately at the present time, this IVF service is limited to women suffering from genetic disorders like Christine and Sue. It would be a wonderful thing if IVF were available on the National Health Service to all who need it. Many women experience severe depression when they cannot conceive a child of the sex they want, and depression can be costly.

A depressed mother may become unable to work or even to look after her family properly. She may then need help in the home and with the children and become financially dependent on the state. Personally, she is condemned to the misery of not being able to bear the normal, mixed family of her expectations. Nobody who has not experienced it themselves can imagine the feeling of helpless frustration when your body produces what you did not intend. It is as if a Rolls Royce car assembly line suddenly produced a Mini. The shock is as great! And worse. With a depressed mother, the whole family suffers.

But this misery is unnecessary. If the method of sex selection described in this book fails for some reason to deliver the desired baby, prudent use of IVF might serve Britain's economy well in the long run, if it could prevent cases of depression. All political parties constantly promote themselves as champions of 'The Family'. Sex selection is a good place to start. Happy mothers make for happy families.

The natural method of sex selection can help to avert depression. The erstwhile happy mother of a planned family of girl and boy, Carole Kitcherside, had a constant yearning for another daughter to fill the void left by the sad death of Claire who died in 1984 of Leucomuscular Dystrophy at the age of four.

I felt as if my whole world had come to an end [wrote Carole]. *My little girl!*

In 1985, we tried again and had another strapping boy, Craig. He was lovely but did not answer my longing for a daughter, which was on my mind constantly. We tried to adopt but with no luck. I could not accept that I would never have a little girl. I grew more and more depressed.

Then a very good friend pointed me to the book, Girl or Boy? Your Chance to Choose. *I bought it and showed it to my husband. We were not sure but we felt we had to try. I followed the girl diet which suited me, as I love milk. I fell pregnant in June 1987. At nine and a half weeks, I went for a Placental Biopsy for Meta Chromatic Dystrophy. The test was positive and I had a termination. They did not tell me the sex of the baby.*

With difficulty, I kept to the timing rules of the method again and repeated the diet. I learned to recognize my temperature drop and my vaginal mucus.

On 16 February 1989, Dominique Claire was born!

I could not believe that after all this time we had a baby girl. It took a while to sink in. At first I was frightened to get too close in case something would happen to her and I would lose Dominique. I have got over that now and I cuddle and love her all day. Dominique will never take Claire's place, but to have a little girl to love again is really wonderful.

I say a big thank you to the book because I, and hopefully other parents, got the chance of having the baby of our choice, instead of leaving it to nature alone.

Carole

There are lucky women who produce a mixed family fortuitously and do not have to expend much thought upon it. However, most females feel deeply about planning their children. And this starts from a very young age. Little girls in my nursery school spent many hours arranging the dolls and teddies into families: 'You can be the big brother. You sit here and look after your little brother. Now, who can be the sister?'

At the risk of being accused of making sweeping statements, I maintain that there is an innate feeling in most females for 'managing' families. It is part of woman's nature to ponder on these things. And this attention continues into adult life when real babies are in question. Most women, if they are honest, will admit to having had at some time a wish to choose their children. And why not? It is the most natural wish in the world.

Women's reasons for choosing are myriad. Some are tragic and some are amusing. Here are a few from the letters I have received.

Many wives say they want a specific sex for someone else in their family. 'A son for my husband in an all girl family' or 'a daughter for my husband [a very popular request]' or 'a granddaughter for Granny who had only sons herself'. Many of us think we know what other people want – and maybe we are right? It is a pretty safe bet that everybody wants what they haven't yet got. Anybody with a long family history of one sex is usually very keen to change the pattern (*see page 96, Chapter 11 and page 123, Chapter 12*).

Some mothers, like Carole above, want to satisfy the aching void left by the sad death of a previous baby. They will never forget the child who died but they long for a replacement to fill the gap left by the loss of their girl or boy.

In 1991, Teresa was the happy mother of two fine boys but she longed for a daughter to complete her family. After careful timing she became pregnant on her thirtieth birthday, at her first attempt for a girl. But the pregnancy went cruelly wrong. Intensive scanning showed brain damage and spina bifida, and the pregnancy was terminated.

> After the post-mortem, I plucked up courage to ask the baby's sex. It was a daughter. My precious daughter, Charlotte! I could not believe how cruel life can be. As if we had not suffered enough. But at least I knew that we could produce a girl after seven boys on our side of the family. We will be using the theory again, although the sex of the baby fades into insignificance in comparison with the need to know I can produce another healthy baby – boy or girl.

In 1993, I received another letter from Teresa.

> This 16 August at 5.26 pm, I gave birth, by Caesarian section, to my second daughter, Rebecca Claire. I came round to hear my husband crying, 'It's a girl! It's a girl!' I still haven't come down to earth yet. We are both delighted with the mixed family I have always dreamed of. The void left by Charlotte is filled and the boys are very protective towards their little sister.

But for some there are less compelling reasons. Katherine wrote:

> We already had a little boy and we thought it would be nice to have a girl. I think, secretly, I wanted to be able to make and buy pretty dresses! My mother-in-law was thrilled when Helen was born, her first granddaughter after seven grandsons.

The wish to choose reaches across the generations. Grannies want to choose too! When Rosie Bentley was born to join her three brothers, her mother, Janet, said, 'My mother didn't stop crying tears of joy for three days.' Rosie was the first granddaughter after five grandsons.

When they become grandmothers, many women fit more easily into the house of their daughter who probably reproduces the sort of home she grew up in. However much they are loved, daughters-in-law are likely to have different ways of doing things. Eighty-year-old Sylvia mused, 'My three sons are fine men and married delightful wives. But whenever I go to visit my grandchildren, I am always a visitor in the house. I wish I had had a daughter!'

Many daughters who have been very close to their mothers want to repeat that happy rapport with their own daughters. 'I want to copy the good relationship I had with my mother,' commented Catherine.

With three sons, Alison wanted, 'An ally and friend against all those males!' Rebecca welcomed her daughter because, 'I won't be in the kitchen alone during rugby games now, I hope'. And Janet 'didn't fancy being swamped by football kits for the rest of her days'. Simona, a close friend of mine, had four sons before I knew her well. They are a brilliant family and now all her sons are at university or in postgraduate jobs. But when they were still at school and playing rugger on most days, their mother grumbled to me over the washing machine, 'I spend my life washing mud!'

Such sentiments gave Gabrielle pause for thought when she embarked on producing a family.

I had particularly wanted a girl and so was delighted when our first-born was a daughter, Laura. We felt we would probably only have two children, mainly because of our ages (I was already thirty-four). And I had felt quite disturbed by the prospect of being the only female in the household should we have two sons – even though my husband is certainly not an MCP nor particularly macho, sporty, etc. I just wanted a daughter without a specific reason, the same way one wants a child – I think very deep-seated feelings are involved here.

The second time, we wanted to have a son for my husband. His reasons were much the same as mine, though in reverse of course. A lone male amongst females! I understood exactly how Andrew was feeling. He was quite happy to try the temperature-taking and timing – at least for a while! We both rejected the diets – the one for a boy looked downright unhealthy, and I was totally unconvinced of any theory behind it. In the event, I fell pregnant in the very first month. The chart suggested that ovulation had taken place by the fifteenth day on which intercourse took place.

Our hoped for son, Maximilian, was born in October. We are delighted to feel our family is so complete. Laura is very taken with her new brother and we are all feeling jolly pleased with ourselves.

Thank you.

P.S. I have lent the book to a friend with two sons. She is trying for a daughter.

Not all the reasons for choosing are analysed so deeply. Some mothers join in this game of sex selection through cool curiosity and a casual interest in seeing if the method really works. Susan wrote, 'I found it interesting to put your theory to the test.' She did, and got her desired daughter immediately.

With three sons and totally convinced she could only conceive boys, Karen read the book and decided to 'give it a go'. She followed the method exactly, in a disbelieving sort of way, refusing to be told the sex after an amniocentesis test given because of her age (37).

'When the time came and I was pushing the baby out, I became quite excited at the thought *maybe* I was having a daughter at last? Then the midwife said the words I wanted to hear, "You have a daughter, a girl!" I screamed.'

So, like most other mothers, Karen really did have a deep-seated longing for a daughter. But she had managed to try for her girl without getting too uptight about it. Such a laid-back approach is excellent for conceiving girls. If the mother gets too wound up and thinks of nothing but baby girls when she goes to bed, her psychological agitation may play havoc with her menstrual cycle and cause her ovulation day to hop around in a bewildering way.

From her own experience, Dr Miriam Stoppard graphically describes the strain of trying desperately to get pregnant. 'Each month I observed my body for signs of menstruation and was hysterical with grief when the period came. I was just as obsessed, just as depressed, as any woman who cannot have children at all. It was only at the end of the year when I forced myself to be more philosophical that conception occurred.'

Although it may seem like demanding the impossible, it is best to approach the whole choice game in a calm and relaxed manner – laced with a bit of humour, if possible! Make love as you did on your honeymoon, concentrating on your husband and forgetting about babies. Girls often turn up unexpectedly when no one is looking. Perhaps they are bashful even before conception!

Such an event happened to Elaine Clarke of Kent. Her life was ruled by football since her two sons had come along to make up an all male family. She had given up all hope of a girl but she still longed for a female companion. Then Elaine read the method and established that she ovulated on Day 18, so she worked out a plan to make love on Days 13 and 15 to get the timing right.

Day 13 happened but Day 15 didn't, due to Match of the Day or something equally exciting. So I didn't expect anything that month. But surprise, surprise! When my period was five days late, I did a pregnancy test and discovered I was pregnant! The scan predicted a girl but I didn't believe it until I held Melissa in my arms.

And Karen Rimme of Liverpool had the right attitude too.

I had two beautiful little boys, Thomas and Joseph, aged seven and six, but I always wished for a daughter. My friend, Alison, had two boys and read your book. She followed the girl diet and plotted her temperature for one year. The result a beautiful baby girl!

Alison gave me the book to read. Well, it was worth a try, but I couldn't be bothered with diet or temperature taking. For six months, I watched my body for signs of ovulation; it seemed that I actually got a pain around the time of ovulation.

With this in mind, we went on holiday and made love five days before ovulation. Then we forgot everything and enjoyed ourselves. Coming home from holiday, I got stomach pains. Could I be pregnant? Sure enough I was! The result a beautiful baby girl! She is two weeks old and I still haven't come down to earth. Lara (named after Zhivago's lover) was such a surprise! The boys just love her and I feel so complete. Thank you Hazel and a big thank you to Colin, my wonderful husband.

Karen

P.S. Alison is lending the book to our other friend who has two boys. Perhaps she will be as lucky?

Tracy and Mark Bilsland wanted to round off their family of two sons and a daughter with another girl so that a perfect balance of the sexes would be achieved.

Well, we did it, and it's all thanks to you, Hazel! We are thrilled with our
perfect family of two boys and two very beautiful little sisters! Rachel was
christened yesterday at seventeen weeks old. She is a real joy; the easiest of
them all. Even so, I worry about her the most – can't be too careful.
We promise you our family is now complete.
  With very best wishes,
    Mark, Tracy, Rob and Ben, Emily and Rachel

The need for a male heir often features large in the monied section of British society. I sent a copy of my original *Girl or Boy?* book to the Prince and Princess of Wales for a wedding present, with a note saying that they would probably not need it, as the recent Royal family seems to have sex selection all sussed out. This century, many royal couples have produced the traditional story-book boy first, followed by a girl, e.g. the Queen and Prince Philip, Princess Margaret and Tony Armstrong Jones, Princess Anne and Mark Phillips. Or were these families just a happy accident?

Whether Charles and Diana read my book I don't know, but they very soon provided two potential heirs to the Kingdom of Great Britain. Perhaps they just wanted to do their duty and be different?

I have had enquiries from wives of wealthy landowners asking for a boy first to provide a son and heir in the traditional way, however archaic and questionable that may be. In some confusion, Suzanne wrote: 'I definitely want our first child to be a son because that will take the pressure off me to produce again in order to bear a son, if the first one wasn't.' In the spring of 1988 her first-born son and heir arrived.

Is not Suzanne's problem reminiscent of the Asian dilemma I referred to earlier? Great pressure, often unspoken, can be brought to bear on a woman in cases of heirship too. The old inheritance practice in England whereby boys inherited but girls did not, is fortunately fading out and inheritance passes to females – monarchical succession is being discussed by the Royal family just as this book is being prepared for publication. Unfair inheritance laws seem an anachronism in our increasingly unisex society, where diplomacy expects fair division between the offspring of both sexes.

In my own family, we as parents help each child as much as we can when individual need arises during our lifetime. But in our Wills, unless something untoward happens, our property and goods will be divided equally among the three, if they survive us. Or among their children, if they die prematurely. I think such fairness is the most peaceable legacy parents can leave. I imagine that in most families it is like this. Difficulty arises when there are great lands and property at stake which are attached to a family name.

In fact, the desire to pass on a family name is important to many people. Sue wrote, 'We have a four-year-old girl and we thought we would try for a boy because my husband wants someone to carry on his surname.'

You may ask, 'What's in a name?' I would answer, 'A surprising amount'. You notice that the author of this book is Hazel Chesterman-Phillips. This is rather a mouthful but I have started attaching my maiden name of Chesterman. As I get older, I come across many instances of lost connections with people who knew me under a different name before I was married.

For twenty years, our garage was the local collecting-point for the recycling of newspapers and a local woman brought her contribution every month to the Phillips' house. Chance had it that we never met on these occasions until we closed down recently in favour of the Council's new collecting-site. At our final collection, I came face to face with Mary who dropped her bundle with the exclamation, 'So it's you! Hazel Chesterman. I never knew!' Mary and I had been in the same year at school.

Six months before he died, I met Dr Roberts in the greengrocer's queue where we chatted. We knew each other on surname terms only. He talked about his former job at the Medical Research Council Centre in Mill Hill and I asked if he knew my brother, who had also worked there in cancer research before he died. He cried, 'Not Freddy Chesterman?' 'Yes. Chesterman is my maiden name.' He had worked with my brother for twenty years and he lived just round the corner from me! But the name-link had been missing and years of friendship were wasted.

So now I am launching a campaign for married women to take on a double-barrelled surname incorporating both their maiden name and their husband's surname. Of course divorce and further marriage would complicate things a little, but names can be changed with husbands.

When they married, my daughters continued to use their maiden name because they wanted to keep their own identity for personal and business reasons. But, since her children have started school, Sheena uses her married name (husband's surname) in all transactions connected with their education, to simplify matters and to put the children at ease with a conventional name like that of most of their peers. Children are not bothered by their mother's wish for identity; Mum is tops anyway! They are happy to carry any name that gives them security – as long as it fits in with everyone else's nomenclature!

However, it might be more generally satisfactory, if double barrelling becomes the norm. In Britain, many professional women just stay Ms Smith or Ms Chesterman or Ms Whatever their maiden name was. But, when writing a book dealing with such intimate details of married life, I felt I should be a Mrs. Hence my lengthy double-barrelled name!

Europe is ahead of us in this matter. Holland already has a similar system of double-barrelling on marriage; and from birth, Russian women have their father's name as a middle name with the suffix 'nya' meaning 'daughter of'. For example, Anna Petrovnya – Anna, daughter of Petrov. On marriage, the husband's name is added: 'Anna Petrovnya Karenina'.

Whatever the merits or demerits of our culture, keeping on a name can be a pressing reason for wanting to choose a son.

So, there is a desire to choose for many reasons: some momentous, some frivolous, most deeply felt and all very natural. These are feelings which many of us have and no one should be ashamed of them.

CHAPTER 6

HOW TO CHOOSE

UNNATURAL SELECTION

For centuries couples have wanted to choose the sex of their children. Theories began in the Ancient World. Aristotle recommended lying on the right side for a boy and on the left side for a girl – in Latin, the word for 'left' is 'sinister'. Did this carry unfair implications for the usually less preferred sex? Various foods were thought to influence the sex – bitter and sour for boys; sweet and sugary for girls. Perhaps the origin of the diet method?

Seventeenth-century aristocrats who wanted a son and heir, started tying up their left testicle and, when that didn't work, they took the drastic measure of actually cutting it off! And to this day, there are innumerable conflicting theories about timing, position and diet.

Certain Ancient Romans had a few ideas too. Around 204 BC, Tiberius Sempronius Gracchus married a wife, Cornelia, and told her, 'I want twelve children of alternate sexes: boy-girl all the way down.' And they did it! Except for one hiccup in the middle when they got two daughters in succession.

To my mind, the best of these theories came from a Greek philosopher, *circa* 350 BC. Empedocles was aware of a link between the timing of intercourse and the sex ratio of babies. He reckoned that the temperature of the womb was of paramount importance in determining the sex of a child. He wrote:

> *Into clean wombs the seeds are poured and*
> *When therein they meet with Cold,*
> *The birth is girls; and boys when*
> *Contrariwise they meet with Warm.*
> *For bellies with warmer wombs become*
> *Mothers of boys.*

(Fragments 65 and 67)

So, Empedocles had the right idea about the importance of the female body's environment. But he was mistaken about the correct criteria for natural sex selection which is what we shall look at later in this book. Hormonal chemical changes in the *woman* favour a particular sex of sperm; warmth in the *man* is significant for the begetting of girls (*see page 56, Chapter 8*).

In the technological twentieth century, Dr Ron Ericsson offered something different. This affable millionaire from the plains of Wyoming drives a car with the number plate: X OR Y, and revels in the name of Mr Sperm! He claims that there are 15,000 'Ericsson' babies in the world, conceived over the last fifteen years through his method of sex selection. Women have flocked to this sympathetic man who emptied their pockets and filled their hearts with happiness.

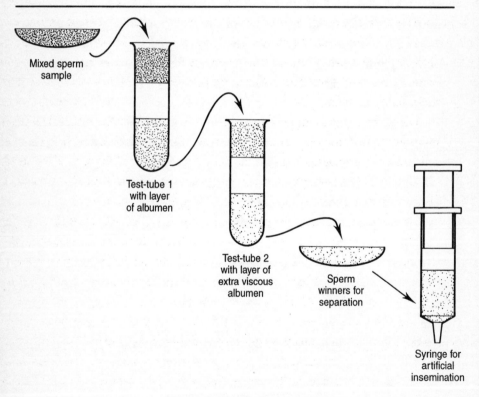

Mixed sperm sample

Test-tube 1 with layer of albumen

Test-tube 2 with layer of extra viscous albumen

Sperm winners for separation

Syringe for artificial insemination

Fig. 8: Sperm Separation

Dr Ericsson invented a method of separating the X and y sperm. As we saw in Chapter 2, each sperm carries either a female X chromosome or a male y chromosome. These carry genetic information which determines the sex of the child. A girl or boy is conceived depending on which sperm penetrates the egg first.

So a key to sex selection is to find a way of separating the male and female sperm and then allowing only one sort to enter the woman's vagina, through artificial insemination in a hospital or surgery. This is what Ericsson claims to have done, with the high percentage success rate of 80 per cent for boys and 70 per cent for girls.

Ericsson's method is to set the sperm on a sort of obstacle course, set to pick only the fittest winners. It is assumed that the male-bearing androsperm swim faster and more aggressively than the female-bearing gynesperm.

A test tube of albumen, a jelly-like substance, is provided for the sperm to swim through. This is meant to handicap the gynesperm (X) leaving the androsperm (y) to reach their goal first. The sperms swim on their own, in active separation. After about one hour, the sperm which have made it to the bottom of the test-tube are collected, and then taken out. This fraction has the better sperm as regards their shape, fertility and progressive motility which is their ability to swim.

The winners are then put into a second test-tube of a physiological solution of known concentration. Then the viscosity of this solution is increased so that only the very strongest sperm get through to the bottom of the second test-tube. These Gold Medal winners, as it were, are then separated, and a sample of androsperm or gynesperm is artificially inseminated into the woman.

Of course, if every stage of this clever method works, there must be 100 per cent success in choosing the sex of the baby, as there are no sperm of the 'wrong' sex involved. And when it works, it brings the delight we saw last year on the faces of the parents of the first successful birth at the London gender clinic: a chosen baby daughter.

'The mechanism, or mechanisms, remain unknown,' says Dr Ericsson. 'We do not know how this method works.' Because of this lack of explanation, many doctors remain sceptical. But 80 per cent is a high success rate, and Dr Ericsson's method still attracts many women whose need has been addressed by his technological method of unnatural sex selection.

In America, Dr Ericsson's method goes by the name of Gametrics Ltd. (You may remember from Chapter 3 that *gamete* is the word for sex cell.) Gametrics Clinics are established in many states of America, and in other countries round the world. In 1991, the patent was bought by Dr Ravindra Gupta in Waltham-stow, East London. He tried to start a clinic but was prevented by medical and legal authorities from opening. In 1993, two North London doctors, Dr Alan Rose and Dr Peter Liu, circumvented the objections and also bought the rights to practise the sperm separation method. Their address is:

The London Gender Clinic
140 Park Road
Hendon
London NW4 3TL
Tel: 0181 202 2900

My first reaction to the arrival of the gender clinic was gladness that there were, at last, some doctors in England who understood the natural and fervent wish in many women to choose the sex of the children they bear. Comprehension of this deep feeling is woefully lacking in most doctors who show little or no sympathy. Indeed, they dismiss the idea of choosing as being something unworthy. Women are often made to feel guilty and wrong for entertaining the very idea.

My doctor was absolutely horrified when I mentioned that I was trying to choose the sex. He said I should be grateful for any baby (which of course I am). He made me feel that I was almost wicked for wanting to choose. It was a most uncomfortable session. I left feeling confused and miserable.

Gillian

I don't know why doctors should take this attitude to one of the most natural longings that most parents have at some time or another. It is reasonable to expect doctors to be primarily concerned with the health and well-being of any child. But what of the mother's mental health? This is precious too, and anything to promote that is surely to be applauded. Prevention is always better than cure, and never more so than in cases of depression. One only has to read my post-bag to see the difference in the mental state of the exhilarated mother who has just given birth to the child of her choice, and the downcast mother who resignedly faces years, albeit staunchly undertaken, of caring for a child she did not completely desire.

Dr Ericsson recognized this need in women and exploited it, to fill parental hearts with contentment. He offered a good chance of getting a chosen child and women responded whole-heartedly. Now, many other doctors are jumping on the bandwagon with hope of similar success. I do not altogether condemn these doctors. They are answering a need that is otherwise ignored and, like most other people, they are using what knowledge they have to make money where possible. Though from the customer's point of view, the fees sometimes seem larger than are fairly warranted. Peony wrote:

The doctor sat us down for half an hour and told us lots of things we knew already about ovulation and testing kits. I could hardly believe it when he asked for £100 at the end of this so-called consultation.

Such is the way of private medicine.

My main objection to these expensive gender clinics is that they create a two-tier system of sex selection. Their sophisticated technology is available only to the rich, but those who are not so well-off may desire a small mixed family just as strongly.

My second reaction to the gender clinics is similar to the official medical opinion in this country. Representatives of the British Medical Association (BMA) expressed concern at so much money changing hands over something that is not yet 100 per cent successful. British doctors, working on this method of sperm separation, say that they will probably not be able to perfect it for another five years.

However, I do not deny that this clever method of sex selection has certain successes. On 15 March 1994, many of us joined in the thrill of congratulations to Gillian and Neil Clark on the birth of Sophie May, the first triumph of the London Gender Clinic. For a mere £650, a sister turned up at last for her two brothers. 'It's just a miracle,' said Mrs Clark and her husband. 'Now our family is complete.'

On the other hand, with three daughters, one of my clients, Miranda, turned to the gender clinic in hopes of a boy. Some months later she wrote to me: 'Three visits and two inseminations cost me £1250. And still I am not pregnant. I have returned to your method, Hazel. Your book is my Bible now.'

Miranda is now the happy mother of a mixed family, complete with her son.

Dr Ericsson admitted to me some years ago that, once the sperm had been raced through his albumen experiment, it was still very difficult to separate them accurately. And more problems lay ahead in getting the woman pregnant. 'Too often the artificial insemination does not work, and my success rate is still slightly lower than yours.'

In 1994, I took part in a Kilroy-Silk chat show debating the practices of the new London Gender Clinic. The plaintiffs in this case were Mr and Mrs Berryman, the parents of five sons. They had withdrawn £2000 of their savings and redundancy money and turned to the gender clinic in final hopes of having a much wanted daughter.

I argued that their all-male family was probably in great part due to their fertile father's high sperm count, as well as to timing. There were unbelieving smiles all round at such a ridiculous suggestion. Nobody had heard of a bias towards boys through a high sperm count, and my strange ideas were laughed into their proper place. The clever technology at the gender clinic would overcome this problem. Treatment proceeded and in October the press made the announcement: To Kenneth and Cheryl Berryman – a sixth son!

The gender clinic takes no notice of the natural timing of sex selection which holds that insemination, whether natural or unnatural, on the day of ovulation produces a boy. But, to better the chances of conception being achieved, artificial insemination is given at the most fertile time of the month: ovulation. So, if the sperm separation is not 100 per cent effective, an androsperm is likely to win the race and a boy will be conceived. This is what gave the cheery Berrymans their great family of fine sons. Sadly, I have since heard from Cheryl that she is being treated for depression. I am so sorry, but not surprised. Even the most recent high technology has not helped her and Kenneth to a daughter. And it hurts, it really hurts, writes Cheryl. She tells me she is considering one final attempt by the natural method.

I wish her well and, when she is ready, will work closely with her to bring her her heart's desire.

As we both live in Mill Hill, I travelled home after this TV programme in a shared car with Gender Clinic's Dr Rose. The latter told me that his colleague Dr Liu had two teenage daughters and had been trying for twelve years to get a son. So far, the sperm separation method had not worked for him. I wrote Dr Liu a letter of sympathy and suggested he might like to try my natural method. I have not heard from him but Dr Rose appreciated the possible irony of the situation!

So much for clever unnatural selection! Let us now consider my alternative method.

NATURAL SELECTION

We have seen how the procedure in the gender clinics is trying to outwit nature with clever technology. And it has some success. My method of sex selection takes a different approach. It is not a matter of *overruling* nature. It is rather a matter of discovering and *obeying* nature's own rules.

We live in a physical world run along regular lines, and I thought there must be a natural law for sex selection, as there is for other physical processes. If we could discover this law, why should we not collaborate with it in choosing the sex of our children? Instead of fighting nature, I would try to discover her rules and co-operate with her.

For many months, I hunted for the natural principles of sex determination. I read as much as I could on the subject, which wasn't a great deal thirty years ago – mostly literature from the Ancient World. I questioned anyone who might be able to advise; and I pumped my relations for any relevant information, which most of them could not remember. But most of all, I considered my own experience as a young mother of three years of marriage and two baby daughters. It was this personal scenario that provided me with a pattern on which to work.

The rules I deduced are very strict, but they are fair. If we follow them exactly, they are honoured and we get the child of our choice. If we make a mistake, we do *not* get what we hoped for. The difficulty is, to comprehend *all* the rules and all the means of conforming to them.

Ever since I first published the idea of being able to choose the sex of a baby, objections have been thrown at me. 'You shouldn't be doing this! You are arrogantly playing God and interfering in nature!' Here is my reasoning: How else can God work but through human hands and minds? If you believe that God set the rules, I do not argue with you. I would follow the old adage: 'God helps those who help themselves.' If we can discover the natural law of sex selection, wherever it comes from, let us learn its dictates and work in harmony with it. Judging from my own experience and from some of the letters I have received, there comes a thrilling sense of satisfaction and well-being when this natural method is tried and followed through to success.

The method seemed so absolutely logical [wrote Maggie, mother of four sons]. *It was worth a try. We found it easy to avoid the middle of the month and we kept to the rules. When our daughter turned up, I found it hard to believe at first. But the euphoria continues from day to day and I never wake from my dream. I feel a strange smugness; the feeling is like a million pounds! Thanks for alerting me to this wonderful method.*

There can be no good reason why we should not try to understand the fascinating way in which our world works. Such discoveries are how a great deal of human comfort has come about. In 1833, Michael Faraday's study of the movement of electrons in a piece of wire led eventually to the discovery of electricity and all the benefits that that has brought to humanity. But it took a lot of hard work and experimentation before electricity was fully understood. Once they *are* understood, natural laws are often elegant in their simplicity. Any difficulty lies in our attempts to follow them precisely.

As to interfering with nature, I would point out that this is what many of us do most of the time. When did you last take an aspirin? When did you last call the doctor? We often use medication to interfere with the insidious infirmities of the natural world. My father was a Specialist in Tropical Medicine and he spent his life interfering with the natural order, or rather disorder, in Africa where people are ravaged by many horrible diseases. I myself am just waiting for someone to interfere effectively with the natural course of multiple sclerosis.

However, I do not see my method of sex selection as *interfering* with nature. As I have said, it is a matter of going along with nature's own rules in harmony and co-operation. Her rules are there for anyone to try. They are the same for princes and paupers the world over.

Some people argue that tampering with nature's rules will have dire effects. What will happen if *all* the Chinese choose to have boys? My first reaction would be one of relief. A period of boys only might do more to solve China's desperate population problem than any number of condoms! A generation without girls would mean a generation of nil population growth.

Admittedly, a scenario where only boys were born might lead to the problem of too many males chasing too few females, as has recently been reported in the newspapers. If this situation gets out of hand, we could speculate that governments might have to resort to an extreme ploy like advocating poly-andry as a temporary measure. But this is unlikely and this sort of change in the mating pool would be spread over a long time; it would not happen overnight. Perhaps it would bring another change too. Girls would soon become highly valued members of the society; something which they have never been so far, in that part of the world.

The female sex would benefit from being more highly esteemed in China. Perhaps one way of helping to right the balance of the sexes would be for the government to offer inducements to couples to produce girls. Alternate years might be designated as 'The Year of the Girl', and Community or National Honours and/or financial rewards offered to couples who chose to bear girls.

I cannot believe that any human society, least of all the astute Chinese, is stupid enough not to right the balance when they see the population balance swinging too much in the boy direction, thus creating a dearth of the other sex. China, being one of the most organized nations on earth as regards social awareness, would no doubt follow the tradition of past leaders like Mao Tse-tung who managed to move this enormous nation in new directions. Eventually, there must come everywhere the recognition that our world is made up of two sexes, and neither can do without the other. Again, co-operation is the golden rule.

If sex selection becomes the norm, it is likely that there will be, especially in Asian and Eastern countries, an initial swing towards boys because of the various religious and social demands of these societies. But ultimately, or even soon, they would probably settle back into a fifty-fifty ratio. My own research supports this view.

Most women want a small mixed family. If they can achieve a mixture of the sexes early, their family will be concluded sooner. Most women who write to me want whichever sex they have not yet got. In the first 5000 letters I received, there was only one request for a repeat of the same sex. This was for reasons of expedience; the house had only two bedrooms and the parents wanted to put both girls in together. But most parents want to experience both sexes in their children. A child of the opposite sex usually rounds off a contented family. The commonest comment in letters announcing the happy arrival of such a child is: 'Now our family is complete!'

This is not to say that single sex families are in any way deficient; I know some first-rate ones. But mothers in particular often feel that they are missing out on something if they have not experienced the full potential of motherhood by having children of both sexes. A mixed family is desirable for many reasons, not least for the sake of variety in the life of the parent who tends the children. A mother must and usually does cherish her child of whatever sex, but the variation of a different gender makes all her work seem novel and fresh. A different sex brings new challenges and new rewards.

In the United Kingdom, we have an official body which regulates sex selection techniques and the use of embryos in artificial insemination. This watchdog is called the Human Fertilization and Embryology Authority (HFEA). In 1993, the HFEA published a Consultation Document on Sex Selection. The comprehensive nature of this compassionately written document covers all aspects of sex selection: medical, social and ethical. Although I do not agree with all their conclusions, I have tried in this book to consider many of the questions raised by the HFEA. Their paper has some salutary warnings on how adults should behave when choosing the sex of their baby. One paragraph which gave me pause for thought was this:

Paragraph 28 *If a couple had children of one sex but would have preferred one of the other, the welfare of the existing children might be affected by the arrival of one of the preferred sex.*

I was so horrified at this thought that I immediately wrote off to Sheena, my elder daughter, to get her opinions from thirty years ago, if she could remember them? This is what she wrote back:

Personally, I think that a child could find the anticipation and arrival of another child of the 'wanted' sex hurtful – could construe it as a feeling that it was not wanted/good enough itself, for example, or not loved as much. Of course, the arrival of a younger sibling is disturbing anyway; parents feel differently towards different children in the same family. Much depends on how everything is handled. In our own family, I always had the feeling (possibly erroneous!), that Mum preferred boys and Dad, girls. But this is not an uncommon set-up and I might well have felt this even if my brother's sex had not been chosen.

So you see, I slipped up a bit here. In my joy at getting the mixed family I wanted, I did not watch my words and behaviour carefully enough. I assumed that a five-year-old would not be thinking about such things. But I should have realized how children listen to adult conversations and pick up the odd dropped remark which can colour their outlook on life.

However, my subsequent 'handling' of the situation must have improved because Sheena and Richard became the best of friends. Later, in their teens, Dick was able to help Sheena over an emotionally sticky patch, and Sheena was a loving support to Dick during a critical illness. These experiences further drew them together and now Sheena's second son bears Dick's name – Matthew Richard.

A final word from my sunny natured second daughter, Penny, who was nearly three when Dick was born: 'I remember coming in to Granny's lounge and feeling excited because everyone looked so happy. And then we all had a lovely tea!'

It is obviously easy to win over two-year-olds! Penny and Dick have always scrapped happily together.

As well as the sex of the child, there is the question of birth order. The traditional fairy-story arrangement of a boy first followed by a girl is still the most popular. I know I dreamed of such a family when I was still at school. I had all sorts of ideas about an older brother's friends providing a ready set of boyfriends for a subsequent daughter. Now older and wiser, I realize what a foolish, old-fashioned notion that was. Many twentieth century girls have a vastly wider mating pool, as the opportunity for jobs and travel arises. And your elder brother's choice of friends is not always yours!

There is a lot to recommend a completely different type of family. It would surely make for a very dull world if all families were tailored the same. Moreover, there is the danger of an undesirable family structure arising. Would we find ourselves with a pattern of pushy, over-ambitious first-born males, followed by meek second-born females? The Warnock enquiry into human fertilization alerted us to this possibility.

It is often suggested that a majority of couples would choose that their first child was male, and if this happened, it could have important social implications, since there is considerable evidence that the first-born siblings may enjoy certain advantages over younger siblings. This would have particular implications for the role of women in society.

But the feedback I've had does not seem to corroborate the likelihood of this occurring. Apart from those under pressure of culture or heirship (*see pages 23 and 25, Chapter 5*), few women want to choose the sex of their first baby – the element of surprise is so exciting! It is when mothers have had two or more of the same sex that they want to be able to choose the other. And if their second child gives them the mixed family that most women want the 'stop-at-two' aim of this book will be greatly enhanced (*see page 166, Chapter 15*).

CHAPTER 7

MY STORY

'I advise against having children,' said the doctor. 'For one in your condition it would not be prudent. Better not take the risk.' He did not elaborate on my 'condition'.

All I knew about my problem was that I had unpredictable bouts of double vision and a gammy right leg which let me down at inconvenient moments. Three years earlier, in the middle of a school tennis match, this leg had suddenly turned into a paralyzed block of wood which wouldn't do what I wanted it to do. I lost four games in a row and dragged myself off the court in confusion.

My father, a doctor who was later knighted for his services to medicine, immediately diagnosed what he had suspected for some time. But out of a spirit of protectiveness, neither he nor his specialist colleagues told me the diagnosis; they fobbed me off with names like 'neuralgia' and 'spasm'. Although I continued to be plagued with problems that affected my eyes and move-ment, it was ten years and three pregnancies later before I learned the truth from a medical student at the Middlesex Hospital.

Expecting my third baby, I was sitting with the other pregnant mums in the antenatal clinic waiting to see the doctor. A student put his head round the cubicle curtains and called out, 'Who is the patient with Multiple Sclerosis?' Nobody moved and he called again. I suddenly wondered, 'Perhaps he means me?' I got up and went to see and there it was written on my notes.

I felt rather a fool not to have guessed. But in those days, not much was known about MS. The Creeping Paralysis, as it was called, was rather hushed up, just as mention of cancer used to be. There were no adverts or articles in magazines as there are today. So, although it might seem a harsh way to find out, I shall always be grateful to that medical student because then I knew what I had to cope with.

In many ways, having a label makes it easier to handle the unbelievable sensations of burning and tingling which come with MS. Formication is the medical term for this sensation because it feels like ants (*formicae* in Latin) running all over you! I sometimes used to think I was going mad with such crazy sensations but, when I knew the name of the disease, I looked it up in the library and learned that, as MS patients go, I was quite normal. Then it became a ludicrous game, trying to deal with each bizarre symptom as it arrived.

I am lucky, because even severe attacks of MS have been followed eventually by a remission and, with the unfailing help of a solicitous husband, I have managed to live a full life, albeit somewhat limited by too many rest periods for my liking! A daily midday siesta became a must for me. I had to cut my life's coat according to the cloth of MS. I recovered enough to go to teacher training college at Homerton, Cambridge, where I met my future husband, then a Classics Scholar, now a London University lecturer in Indonesian language and literature. We married a year later and our family soon followed.

Then I understood the advice of the doctor who warned me against the stresses of motherhood. After each birth I had a relapse and had to stop breast feeding because I could not hold the baby to the breast for long. Although during pregnancy I had felt fine. This doctor was only going by the light of his time when MS was feared, and not understood as it is today. And there are sad cases where his advice is valid. If MS hits you hard and life becomes cruel, there is nothing you can do apart from sitting like patience on a monument and trying to smile at grief as much as you can. But for those like me who have what is known ironically as 'benign' MS, life does not have to stop with the onset of the disease. We just have to change gear and slow down in accommodation. 'We must adapt to survive,' said Charles Darwin, referring to all living creatures. And this truth holds especially for those with MS.

When I was forty, I was forced in to a frustrating 'adaptation' period. A severe attack of MS left me sitting helplessly on the floor, unable even to crawl around much. I got sick of sitting on my monument. Then I had a brilliant idea! Something I could do on the floor was read books. I would read books as long as my eyes would let me. I would learn a bit about my pet subject of sex determination. I would take a degree with the Open University!

I can't recommend this sort of activity enough to MS patients when they are badly struck by the disease. There are so many interesting courses to choose from; from Baby and Child Care to Nuclear Physics. You do not have to study for a full degree and you can take your time over whatever interests you. It took me ten years to get my degree in Science and Philosophy (neither of which I had touched before). But during that time, with the help of the brilliant TV physics programmes, I mentally travelled to outer space and back; I studied biology and did chemistry experiments; I delved into the inner places of the brain and I learned the physiology and philosophy of life and death – and sex selection.

And all from my cushion on the floor! Try it. Studying with the Open University can be a great source of new interests when the kids are almost grown up and beginning to leave home. And inactive MS patients may need it more than most.

Whether to have children or not if you have MS depends a great deal on your personal circumstances and the help you will be able to get from grannies, aunts, sisters, friends and the social services. Personally, I was blessed with a very fit and devoted mother and her sterling housekeeper, 'Mrs B', who lived quite near. I could always count on them in an emergency when my usually dependable husband was at work or away. This sort of back-up makes a great difference to a mother with MS. Child rearing can be very hard for you, and your husband, if you are on your own and not in full health. I have heard from other MS mothers to the same effect. 'My mother is a God-send,' reported Karen on the phone.

With this sort of support, I rebuffed the kind doctor who counselled me against having children. 'Of course I shall try for children! I have just got engaged to my future husband and we couldn't contemplate not having a family.' The doctor bowed his head, 'Well, if you must, have them quickly while you are still young.'

My elder daughter must have been listening! Sheena arrived earlier than we planned, less than a year after we were married. And her conception led to the beginning of this book. So willy-nilly, I took the advice given me by the older, experienced physician and had all my children within five years. Looking back, I am very grateful for that warning from the doctor, because MS does not often stand still for long and I don't think I would have been able to cope with motherhood in later life. Now, I stand aghast at the energy and efficiency demanded of my daughters in coping with their young. As regards the progression of my MS: at fifty-five I reached the top of the proverbial hill of life, fell down and broke my hip and careered down the other side rather fast into a wheelchair where I have been mostly ever since. Sadly, I had to give up the nursery school I had run in my home for twenty-five years in favour of something more sedentary. Fortunately, I moved on to the fascinating job of answering thousands of letters from enterprising women thirsting to choose the sex of their children. And this is how I chose mine.

Sheena was conceived after intercourse on 19 November 1957. I know the exact date because that was the only time just after our wedding that we didn't use contraception. We mistakenly thought we were in the 'safe' period because it was only the fifth day of my cycle, as soon as I had finished menstruating. Furthermore, we had not been married very long and I naively thought that 'pregnancy wouldn't happen so quick' (to quote a letter I received recently from Rabinder). But once is enough with a young, fertile couple. I conceived. And we had – a girl. One of the best mistakes we ever made! 'Good,' said my mother. 'She will soon grow up to give you a hand.' Which she did!

Two years later, we wanted another child and I thought, 'Well, I seemed pretty fertile on the fifth day of my cycle. That seems to be when we can produce babies.' So we repeated the procedure exactly and got – another girl! In spite of my willing and praying for the opposite. My first word on the delivery table was, 'Bother!' Another mistake which has given us pleasure ever since! And Penny's conception established the germs of my growing ideas about sex selection.

After this, I began to think. I wanted a mixed family. Both times I had had a girl and both times intercourse had been on the same day of my cycle. Could these two facts be related? Did the sex of the child depend on the relation between the time of intercourse and the time of ovulation?

Admittedly, I was working on a completely unscientific hunch, but the more I thought about it the more I was convinced that this must be the crux of the matter. Sex determination must be dependent on the day in the menstrual cycle on which intercourse took place. Of course, conception itself can only occur when the woman has ovulated and released an egg.

Knowing that the male species were the more powerful of the sexes but that the females were more long-lived and tenacious of life, I wondered if this rule held for the male y-carrying androsperm and the female X-carrying gynesperm even before conception.

It is known that the longer tailed androsperm are the faster swimmers and that environmental conditions in a woman's body are most favourable to sperm on the day of ovulation. So, with intercourse on this peak day, the speedier males would win the race to the egg and a boy would be conceived.

But if intercourse took place some days before ovulation when conditions were less favourable, the androsperm would die off within a few days, but the the more enduring gynesperm would survive better while waiting for the egg. As soon as it appeared at ovulation, one would be waiting ready to fertilize it. Hence a girl would be conceived. Females are crafty even before conception!

Therefore we decided that, in the hope of conceiving a boy next time, we would reverse our procedure. Instead of trying early in the cycle, we would aim for intercourse and conception on the day of ovulation.

So I set about pin-pointing my day of ovulation, fourteen days before the next period. The only method available then was temperature taking. Ovulation occurs when there is a mid-month drop in temperature followed by a sharp rise. Every morning for six months, I took my temperature before getting out of bed in the morning after my main sleep of the night. (This is the basal body temperature, when you are at your most relaxed.) I was careful to keep the thermometer in my mouth for three minutes and I kept a record of the readings. At the end of that cycle, I plotted the readings on to a graph and joined them up to make an easily recognizable pattern (see page 62, Chapter 8).

I soon realized that at ovulation I always experienced a slippery, stretchy, jelly-like discharge from the vagina like the raw white of egg. This helped me to plot my chart and determine my exact cycle which was twenty-four days from the start of one period to the start of the next. I was able to identify my ovulation on the tenth day after starting a period.

Having established this beyond doubt, we thought about our next child. Because barrier methods of contraception are not one hundred per cent reliable and because I wanted to give my theory every chance of producing a boy, we abstained from sex that month until the tenth day of my cycle. At midday on Day 10, I again experienced the slippery vaginal discharge and we made love that night. To make conditions perfect for a boy, we made sure that I had an orgasm before my husband although, at that time, I didn't know the full scientific implications of this (see page 58, Chapter 8). I conceived. And felt wretchedly nauseous for the next three months. I never doubted the outcome – a boy!

So the method worked for me, and I revelled in it! There is a certain 'knowledge by acquaintance', as the philosopher Bertrand Russell called it, that only comes through firsthand experience. When my son was conceived, I just knew that I had hit upon the right rule. Somehow I felt it in my body and I never doubted for a moment that my daughters' brother was on his way. Nine months later, when the mid-wife said, 'And he's a bouncing boy!', even though exhausted from a long and tiring labour, I heard myself saying in confident delight, 'I know. I always knew!'

Over the past thirty years, other women have said the same thing to me: 'I sort of felt it in my bones!' I know that reason says you can't be sure of the outcome until the baby arrives, but instinctively I felt I was on the right track. Women's intuition? If you are content to be unscientific. However, this is not a universal truth. Sometimes the desired child comes with the shock of a bombshell:

> *Right from the start, I was sceptical* [wrote Nancy]. *With three boys already, a daughter was not for the likes of us. We kept to the timing; we kept all the rules; but I was sure nature would have the last laugh on us. And she certainly tried! Our baby came out back to front so that even at the moment of birth you couldn't see the sex. My husband said gloomily, 'Here we go again with our football team.' Then the mid-wife turned the baby over and cried, 'Look! He's a girl!'*

I feel that there is nothing as convincing as experience. Successful mums like Nancy have something that even Dr Ericsson's prowess can't match. My son's birth did not come as a surprise to me. Rather, it was the confirmation of one of nature's unveiled maxims.

I spent the next few years bringing my children up and spreading my ideas of sex selection to anyone interested. Soon after Dick's birth, we all went to stay with my husband's sister, Rosemary, in Cheltenham. She was also the mother of two daughters, Julia and Joanna. One day, we were sitting on the lawn playing with the babies, when Rosemary suddenly sighed, 'You lucky thing! With a boy! I wish we could have one too.' I replied, 'It's easy! I'll tell you how.' A year later, Rosemary and Ron's son, Roger, was born.

And this year, 1995, thirty years later, Roger sent news from his home in France that the rule had worked again for him and his wife, Cheryl. On 12 September, son Sam arrived as planned to join his sister, Beth, and made the wanted pigeon pair family. Thus the knowledge is passed on from generation to generation.

In the next forty births among close friends and relations who followed the rules, there was 100 per cent success in choosing the sex of the baby. These births included a girl and a boy born to a woman who, for medical reasons, underwent Artificial Insemination by the Husband (AIH). This procedure took place under highly clinical conditions and the days were carefully chosen by the mother to ensure one baby of each sex.

It was suggested that I write my method down, as many people might be interested. This I did, in a small booklet just containing the rudimentary rules of the method. The journalist Tessa Hilton read this booklet and wrote it up for *Mother & Baby* magazine. Through this publication's wide circulation from London to New Zealand, the method travelled to many countries. Readers who were keen to choose a particular sex of child were invited to act as guinea pigs and put the theory to the test.

Meanwhile, I went on reading as much as I could find on this subject and was delighted to discover that a number of doctors around the world held the same theories and were doing similar research. For instance, half-way across the world, an Indian doctor in Delhi, Dr Inderjit Kaur Barthakur, had been deep in similar research since the 1960s. She had also produced a booklet on sex determination. I corresponded with her.

A year later, the results of couples who had tried the method started coming back. And it turned out that the theory which had worked for me was working for over 80 per cent of other families too. The fascinating feedback received from these willing helpers was the basis of my book: *Girl or Boy? Your Chance to Choose,* written jointly by me and Tessa Hilton.

With such a growing sample, it was inevitable that the success rate should fall a bit. To have the method in print was an ambiguous advantage: it was open to everyone to try, but this brought a snag – people read the printed word in many different ways. They bring their own thoughts and wishes to bear on what they read, and sometimes accuracy flies out of the window! 'It was *nearly* the right day!' wailed Linda, after trying unsuccessfully for a boy. But nearly is not good enough when dealing with the preciseness of nature.

Among the group of people who I have been able to interview or otherwise meet face to face (so that I could ascertain that they really understood all aspects of the theory) the success rate has been 98 per cent over the last thirty years. Does this say something about the clarity or otherwise of my writing? Or perhaps 2 per cent is a reasonable failure rate?

Girl or Boy? Your Chance to Choose deals with the correct timing of intercourse in the woman's menstrual cycle. After that was published, I began researching into the man's contribution to sex determination: sperm count. This proves to be highly significant and can even override the timing factor sometimes. Since I have been sending out papers containing this knowledge, the success rate is creeping up again. Among readers who have notified me, it currently stands at 83 per cent.

Many people say to me, 'Ah! but only the successful mothers write back to you.' Of course, this is a possibility, and I can imagine parents tossing the book away in disgust if the method does not appear to work for them. But this is certainly not one hundred per cent the case. Most unsuccessful women write back in the hopes that, between us, we may get it right next time in true Thomas Kuhn style (*see page 149, Chapter 14*). And they often do!

Many people, unknown to me, get the child they want by reading the rules in my book or in a magazine. Recently, I went to John Lewis' in Brent Cross shopping centre and began chatting to the shop assistant as she measured out my order.

'What children do *you* have?'

'Oh! Two girls – and I've just got a boy.'

'That's very clever of you. How did you manage it?'

'Well, I bought this book by Hazel Chesterman-Phillips . . .'

'Oh – pleased to meet you. I *am* Hazel.'

She gave a yelp. And rushed off to find the manager (poor chap!) to introduce him to me.

Progressing to the other end of Brent Cross, I chatted in similar vein to the salesgirl in Fenwick's who said, 'I know all about *you*. I used your method to get my son.'

However, now that the book is in many languages, I have unfortunately lost track of people's experiences world-wide. I should dearly like someone or some clinic to help me run a scientific investigation of my method of sex determination. I think that the enterprising women who practise this method so painstakingly could demonstrate a natural rule for sex selection.

Thus, like many others, we achieved our mixed family – Sheena, Penny and Dick, who grew up to do us proud by each winning scholarships to Cambridge or Oxford. I wait with interest to see what *their* families will be? Will they follow the method set out in the next chapter?

POSTSCRIPT

As I write this, the postman has just dropped in a letter from Karen (*see page 49 of this chapter*).

Dear Hazel

I hope you remember me. I have MS, and I kept writing to you that I wanted to try for a baby girl. I did all that you advised, got pregnant and then had a miscarriage [see page 105, Chapter 11]. I let you know about this the last time I wrote to you.

Well, I got pregnant again after the miscarriage as soon as I could. We did everything you'd said and on 11 July 1995, after an induction two weeks early due to eclampsia, we got our baby girl. And I still can't believe she is actually here. All the nurses kept laughing at me; they'd find me crying and ask why, and all I kept saying was I must be dreaming. I'm so happy; I'm crying now while writing this. I feel I'm the luckiest person in the world. The nurses had to take her off me one night in hospital because I just cuddled her and couldn't stop looking at her, and I wasn't getting any sleep. It is so perfect now we've got two boys and now Jessica Elizabeth. We are all complete. Thank you so much for all your help.

Now I have an MS relapse [as I did each time after the exhausting experience of giving birth] and I can't go out with her, but I just look forward to the relapse passing. I don't care – she's worth every bit; I'd do it all again for her. Hazel, you did make my wildest dream come true.

We hope to hear from you soon,

Karen and Richard

Congratulations to you all! I am so glad Jessica Elizabeth finally turned up as she should. I trust Richard and your mum will be able to cope, with the help of Morecambe's good social services. I hope you will all be carried through by the pleasure of Jessica's arrival. And all too soon, she will grow up to be a help to you. Enjoy your perfect family!

Hazel

CHAPTER 8

THE NATURAL METHOD

Natural sex selection depends mainly upon two components, one from each partner.

1 The woman must arrange the correct timing of intercourse in her menstrual cycle.

2 The man must adjust his sperm count to the required level.

When these two necessary conditions are fulfilled, intercourse usually leads to the conception of a child of the chosen sex.

IN BRIEF

IF YOU WANT A GIRL

MAN   The genitals should be kept warm in close-knit Y-fronts and trousers on the tight side (to lower the sperm count).

WOMAN   Ovulation day should be identified as described in Chapter 9. If possible, hold back from orgasm to maintain the acid environment which favours the gynesperm.

BOTH   To lower the sperm count, have frequent (every other night), unprotected sex as soon as the period finishes until three days (or more, if the man is very fertile) before ovulation. Then stop; or use a barrier method of contraception for the rest of that cycle. If

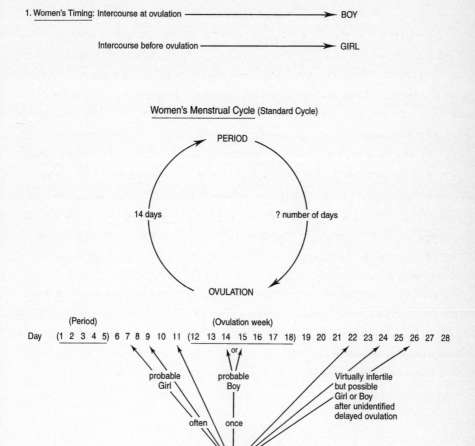

1. Women's Timing: Intercourse at ovulation ⟶ BOY

Intercourse before ovulation ⟶ GIRL

Women's Menstrual Cycle (Standard Cycle)

PERIOD

14 days

? number of days

OVULATION

(Period)   (Ovulation week)

Day   (1 2 3 4 5) 6 7 8 9 10 11 (12 13 14 15 16 17 18) 19 20 21 22 23 24 25 26 27 28

or

probable   probable   Virtually infertile
Girl   Boy   but possible
                                       Girl or Boy
                                       after unidentified
                                       delayed ovulation

often   once

INTERCOURSE

(But see the warning for very fertile fathers of sons on page 58, Chapter 8)

2. Man's Contribution: High sperm count ⟶ BOY

Low sperm count ⟶ GIRL

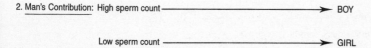

Fig. 9: Sex Determination

conception does not occur after three months of trying, gradually creep up, one day per month, nearer to ovulation. But not too near or you will get another boy! Do NOT make love if you have any sign of the slippery ovulatory mucus. (For possible use of a jock-strap, see p 84.)

With very fertile men who have sons already, as much time as possible, compatible with getting pregnant, should elapse between intercourse and ovulation, to give plenty of time for the male-bearing androsperm to die off before the egg appears at ovulation. (*I conceived both my daughters after intercourse 5 days before ovulation.*)

If you do not fall pregnant immediately, don't worry. Continue to persevere for some months. It is often hard to conceive a girl deliberately because you have to *avoid* the most fertile time of the month at ovulation. If you make love too far in advance of ovulation, you will be outside your fertile time and conception won't occur. If you make love too near ovulation, you risk another boy. You need to be as patient as Nurse Isabel Audley who waited 8 months to get her daughter (*see page 96, Chapter 11*). But she says it was worth the wait! And pregnancy usually occurs much sooner than that.

Finally, see Specific Instructions (*page 61 of this chapter*).

IF YOU WANT A BOY

MAN   The genitals should be kept cool in boxer shorts and loose trousers, allowing cool air to circulate round the testicles.

WOMAN   Ovulation day should be identified as described in Chapter 9. If possible, have an orgasm before your husband; when a woman reaches orgasm, she releases some alkaline fluid which favours the androsperm.

BOTH   To keep the sperm count at a high level in the month in which you want to conceive, abstain from intercourse until the woman *has* ovulated or, if the cycle is too long for such restraint, for at least a week before trying for your son. Wait for the slippery, ovulatory vaginal mucus and then make love *once* while the sperm count is high.

If pregnancy does not occur within three months, check with your doctor as to why you are not conceiving.

Men who know that their sperm count is low may be helped by a course of cold sponging (*see page 82, Chapter 10*).

REASONS FOR THE RULE OF HIGH OR LOW SPERM COUNT

The male-bearing androsperm may be faster swimmers but they do not cope so well with the hazards of the vagina as do their female-bearing gynesperm sisters. Because so many androsperm die off when they are ejaculated into the woman's body, a higher number of them would provide a greater chance statistically of one of their number surviving until it reaches its goal and fertilizes the egg. Hence the need for a high sperm count to beget boys.

The converse of low sperm count follows for the begetting of girls. Because the gynesperm are more long-lived, their number does not diminish so drastically and many will survive even in a low sperm count. Hence a low sperm count can beget girls.

REASONS FOR THE RULES OF TIMING (VERY SIMILAR TO MY HUNCH!)

Conception can only occur at or after ovulation when the egg breaks out of the follicle in the uterus and enters the Fallopian tube. At ovulation, the vaginal environment becomes bathed in alkaline mucus in which both sorts of sperm are viable: the female-bearing gynesperm and the male-bearing androsperm. But the faster swimming androsperm are more likely to win the race to the egg after intercourse on the day of ovulation. Hence a boy will be conceived.

However, at other times of the menstrual month, the vaginal environment is usually acid. Most androsperm cannot survive long in acid, but the hardier gynesperm can live in the woman's body for up to five or six days. So, if intercourse takes place some days before ovulation, the less hardy androsperm will die off before the egg is released at ovulation. But some gynesperm can wait around until the egg appears for them to fertilize. Hence a girl will be conceived.

My doctor read these rules and said incredulously, 'Is that all it is? Ovulation for a boy; before ovulation for a girl? How very simple!' It is this simplicity that convinces me that the method is sound. The basic laws of nature often turn out to be simple, once discovered. As the fourteenth century Occam's razor says, 'Entities are not to be multiplied beyond necessity.' That is, the simplest hypothesis is always to be preferred.

I recommend that women trying for a certain sex of child limit their intercourse that month to what they judge to be the 'right' days. Then stop! In this way, there is no possibility of any sperm getting through to the egg at the wrong time.

Where is the scientific proof of this method? And why does it not work for everyone? I am of the opinion of the great scientist, Albert Einstein, who said, 'Find the answer first and let the proof come afterwards.' Proof of the method described in this book is very hard to come by. I allow that it cannot be proved according to acceptable scientific criteria because I can never observe the final experiment! But I proved it to myself when my own son was born and I concede that the only public proof at the moment is results.

And this is where my readers come in. By exactly following the rules to stack the odds in favour of conceiving the child of your choice, proof will finally come through the weight of numbers of successful parents. Dr Martin Patel rang enthusiastically from King's Cross, London WC1, 'I am recommending more women to you. Your method works, you know. It really works!'

To achieve this success, two hurdles in particular have to be surmounted.

For women, the day of ovulation must be carefully determined and for men, the level of sperm count must be adjusted. We shall consider these hurdles in the next chapters.

SUMMARY

Get the timing *and* the sperm count right, and the child of your choice should turn up.

SPECIFIC INSTRUCTIONS FOR A GIRL

When you are ready to conceive your daughter:
1 The man's genitals should be kept warm in close-knit underpants or a jock-strap, by day only, for *five days* during or after the period.
2 Have free intercourse without contraception, every other night, up until 5 days before ovulation. (If conception does not occur, gradually creep up, in subsequent months, until 4, 3, 2 days before ovulation.)
3 Then stop; or use barrier contraception for the rest of that menstrual cycle. If conception does not take place, repeat the method another month.

Warning! The jock-strap should not be worn for more than *five days*, by day only. More use may temporarily lower the sperm count too much to achieve pregnancy at all. If not pregnant after two months, stop using it (*see page 84*).

SPECIFIC INSTRUCTIONS FOR A BOY

When you are ready to conceive your son:
1 The man's genitals should be kept cool in boxer shorts or underpants and loose trousers.
2 Abstain entirely from sex until the woman has ovulated or, if you have a long cycle, for at least a week prior to ovulation.
3 When the slippery, ovulatory vaginal mucus is present, make love *once* while the sperm count is high.

Men with a known low sperm count may be helped by cold sponging of the genitals. Daily cold sponging or showering should ideally continue for 3 months prior to trying for a boy as 70 days is the duration of spermatogenesis. This would give the sperm a boost from their very beginning. It would also be a test of heroism for the man! But, if it causes pain or discomfort, stop it.

HELP AND HINDRANCE IN FOLLOWING THESE RULES

HELP

There are many gadgets on the market to help you find your ovulation day. These can be very useful to women who find it hard to pin-point this crucial event.

Temperature Charts: available from most chemists, either singly or booklets. 1995 price at Boots – 90p for ten. These are published by G.H. Zeal Ltd, Lombard Road, Merton, London SW19 3UU Tel: 0181 542 2283/6. These charts are clear and easy to follow. But any fertility chart will do.

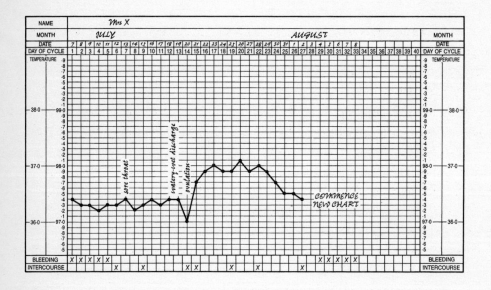

Fig. 10: Example of ZEAL Fertility Chart

Fertility Thermometers: available from most chemists; also from G.H. Zeal Ltd, as on previous page. These are easier to read than the old clinical thermometers because they give the temperature markings in larger divisions which are easier for early morning bleary eyes to focus on!

Electronic Digital Thermometers: There are many digital thermometers on sale today from chemists. They are much quicker and easier to read than the old mercury thermometers. You do not have to keep them in your mouth for so long. Digital thermometers flash your temperature on to a small display panel on the shaft of the instrument for you to read and record. It is simple to plot a chart from such readings.

The Electronic Gadget, Ovin: which I used to confirm my ovulation day, is unfortunately *no longer available*. Its inventor, Dr Michael Ash, sadly died of old age last year after a long life devoted to helping women all over the world to plan their families and practise birth control. His work may have been a precursor of the modern Ovulation Kits which I recommend instead (*see page 78, Chapter 9*). I found Clearplan the simplest to use. BUT, read the instructions carefully and take note of my warning.

Douching: This is an old fashioned aid to sex determination which some grandmothers of my day still recommended. However, I personally did not bother with it; if you get the timing right, your hormones provide the desired environment for you.

What exactly is a douche? A douche is a jet of liquid directed into the body from a pipe. In sex selection, a douche means washing the vagina with a liquid aimed at increasing the acid or alkali environment as required.

An acid douche, for girls, is made up of:
2 tablespoons of white vinegar (acetic acid) in 2 pints of water.

An alkaline douche, for boys, is made up of:
2 tablespoons of bicarbonate of soda in 2 pints of water.
(Let this douche stand for 15 minutes before use, to make sure all the soda is completely dissolved.)

Mary said her doctor had recommended plain yoghurt for an alkaline douche. But beware! I once gave plain yoghurt from Sainsbury's a pH test with litmus paper which immediately turned red, denoting acid! You would have to be very sure that the yoghurt *was* alkaline, and not contaminated with any acid fruit flavouring or preservative. Plain alkaline yoghurt would seem a good idea because it has a thick consistency which would effectively coat the vaginal walls – but make sure that it is alkaline with a pH number more than 7, thus turning litmus paper blue. The bicarb douche might be safer.

Douching applicators are hard to come by now. Only a few posh chemists sell disposable douches and these already contain douching liquid (sterilized or scented water?). But any clean plastic jug with a spout would do as an applicator. You should NOT DRINK a douche; it is strictly for washing the genital area. And always be careful to avoid infection by keeping all douching appliances scrupulously clean.

Personally, I have never used a douche, but I imagine you just lie back in an empty bath or on your bed (on some towelling) and squirt or pour the liquid into the vagina just before intercourse. 'The vinegar douche is a real turn-off!' said Amanda. 'We gave it a miss after a few goes.' However, it seems that you can be quite casual about it and any sort of applicator will do. Sally, a former nurse, who produced a daughter successfully after using an acid douche, told me, 'I just sat on a bidet and sloshed the douche mixture around me, occasionally directing it up the vagina with a horse syringe.'

If you haven't got a bidet or a horse-syringe, a clean washing-up bowl and a jug will do!

The use of a douche inexpertly applied could be uncomfortable and even dangerous because of possible infection (see Wendy Cooper, *The Fertile Years*, p.48).

Position for Intercourse: This can be altered to favour the desired sperm's chances in the race to fertilization. Although again, I did not bother.

Shallow penetration for a girl – face to face missionary position. So that the deposited sperms do not escape the acid environment of the vagina.

Deep penetration for a boy – the rear animal style position. So that the sperms are deposited in the highly alkaline region of the cervix.

There are conflicting views about the value of these two latter precautions: which intercourse position provides the more effective penetration is open to doubt. I only know definitely of one woman who followed this rear position to conceive her boy successfully. I, like Debby (*see page 115, Chapter 12*) conceived both sexes after intercourse in the missionary position.

And, unless you can make a joke of them, both these latter activities may increase the stress of the situation, which is not desirable.

HINDRANCE

Celia wrote:

> My husband is a salesman and is frequently away for stretches of time. When
> he comes home, it is lovely. Like a honeymoon all over again. But sometimes,
> it is not very convenient for temperature charts and timing. If it is the wrong
> day for intercourse, what can I do?

A lot of women find themselves in this predicament. I think the best thing to do
is to have a contraceptive cap handy to use if it isn't the right day for intercourse.
(Your husband need not know anything about it, if you are cleverly discreet.) Be
relaxed about the whole matter and don't limit sex by the calendar! That would
be another turn-off!

CHAPTER 9

FINDING OVULATION

'What exactly *is* ovalation?' asked Trixie.

There is no such thing as *ovalation*! Ovulation with a 'u' is derived from 'ovum': the Latin word for 'egg'. Ovulation is the moment in the menstrual cycle when the ovum bursts out of the follicle in the woman's ovary and enters the Fallopian tube, where it may be fertilized and become, eventually, a baby (*see page 6, Chapter 1*). Ovulation usually occurs 14 days before the next period because this is the time the egg takes to travel down the Fallopian tube from ovary to uterus (womb). Though, as we've seen, this time is variable from woman to woman and also from cycle to cycle. If the egg is *not* fertilized, it will come away from the body in the next period.

Pin-pointing ovulation is a crucial factor for the natural method of sex selection. Hormones change the chemical environment of a woman's body during her cycle, and different times of the menstrual month favour either the X or the y sperm in their race to the egg. As we have seen, the timing method of sex determination depends on the relationship of intercourse to ovulation. Hence the importance of accurately discriminating when ovulation occurs.

This is often the trickiest part of the whole procedure and causes many problems. But nearly all women can be helped by using some or all of the ways described in this chapter. We will start at the beginning, with the menstrual cycle.

The diagram overleaf depicts the standard menstrual cycle of 28 days with ovulation on Day 14, fourteen days before the next period. If you menstruate as regularly as this, you can determine your ovulation by merely counting the days. Personally, I was lucky and had a regular cycle, albeit shorter than the standard 28 days. I menstruated every 24 days with ovulation occurring regularly on Day 10, which was fourteen days before my next period.

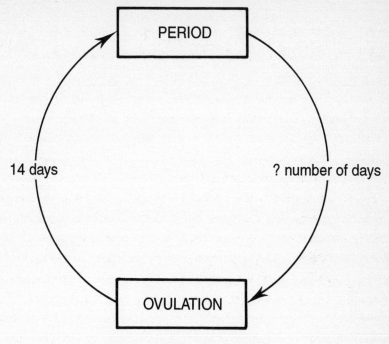

Fig. 11. The Menstrual Cycle

However, many women deviate from this set pattern which sometimes makes distinguishing when ovulation occurs a problem. Certain women ovulate eight or ten days before the next menstruation or some other unusual number of days. There are variations from woman to woman and variations in the same woman from cycle to cycle. Every woman has her own rhythm and must gauge it for herself by watching her temperature and vaginal mucus.

When attempting to work out cycles and days of ovulation, a clear distinction should be drawn between calendar months and menstrual months. The date of the calendar month is irrelevant; its only secondary value is to give information about where you are in the calendar year. But all counting of days should be based on the menstrual month. 'Cycle' is a better word to use because it sometimes runs for less or more than a calendar month. A menstrual cycle runs from the beginning of one period to the beginning of the next. The first day of bleeding (or spotting) counts as Day 1.

If the length of cycles is randomly irregular, a few months should be spent in trying to find some sort of pattern. For example:

Alternately long and short?

Two long, then one short?

Three short, then one long?

If you have the time and skill to make them, bar charts illustrate clearly the regularity or otherwise of your cycles. Such a pattern can be recorded on a simple bar chart like the one below. This will help the woman to gauge more accurately when ovulation is likely to occur.

Sally was having infertility treatment. She had a laparoscopy and then 'conceived a boy very quickly after intercourse at ovulation'. But when thinking about trying for her girl, she found her cycles very irregular. 'Which makes prediction difficult,' she wrote, 'some ovulation days being up to three days on either side of the average.'

The computer buff, Sally, monitored her cycles over two years, and recorded them on the impressive computer bar chart opposite.

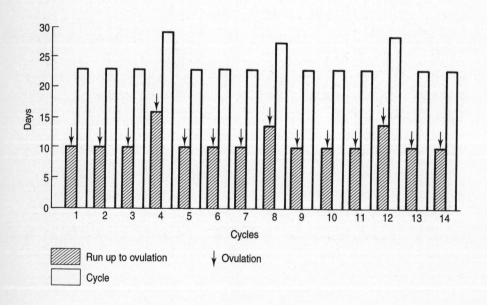

Fig. 12: Bar Chart Showing Menstrual Cycles and Ovulation

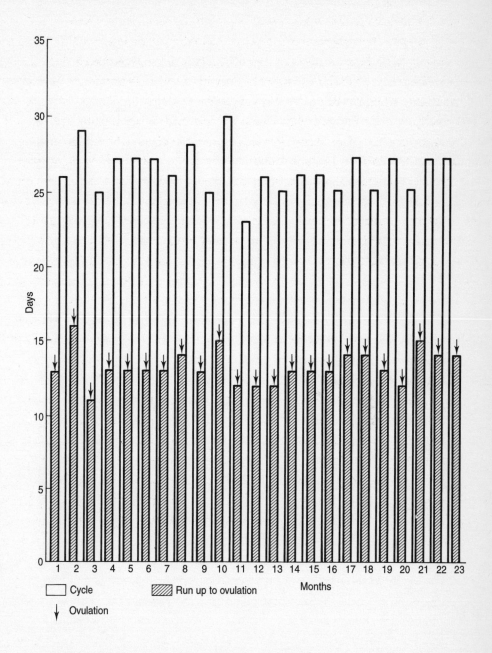

Fig. 13: Computer Bar Chart Showing Ovulation and Cycles Over 2 Years.

This demonstrates how irregular her cycles are, but it also shows clearly that most ovulation days fall on Days 11 or 12. I advised Sally to take these shorter cycles as her criterion. If she stopped unprotected intercourse on Day 8, she would be well before ovulation even in her shorter cycles and wouldn't be caught out by ovulation arriving sooner than expected. And if she *did* happen to be in a longer cycle then, she just wouldn't get pregnant that month. If in doubt, it is always safest to work by the shortest cycle to start with. If you don't get pregnant after three months' trial, creep up nearer to expected ovulation, one day at a time.

Women with very long cycles should monitor them and see if the temperature level changes about fourteen days before the next period. This is a somewhat daunting chore. But it *can* be done usually, with repeated monitoring of cycles. Personally, I don't know how to make such professional-looking computer charts as Sally's, but modest hand-drawn ones like Fig. 19, page 106, serve the purpose adequately.

Normally, ovulation can be ascertained by various physiological methods such as temperature-taking, personal indications and observation of vaginal mucus. There are also ovulation kits available from chemist shops, which monitor the amount of Luteinizing Hormone (LH) in the urine and give useful warning of ovulation (*see page 78, of this chapter*).

Temperature Method Basal body temperature is recorded when the body is at its most relaxed. It can be taken first thing in the morning or whenever the woman wakes from her main sleep of the 24-hour day. Then her bodily metabolism is at its lowest level. The temperature should be taken at the same time each day before any food, drink or activity that would alter the reading. It is best for the thermometer to be put in immediately on waking. Gentle dressing would not disturb the temperature but no exercising or strenuous physical activity should take place. The thermometer should be left in the mouth for five minutes or, if the temperature is taken vaginally or rectally, three minutes should be allowed.

Basal body temperature is usually between 36.2 and 36.3C (97.2 and 97.4F). It may be a bit higher during menstruation but the chart should begin on Day 1 of the cycle, i.e. the first day of the period. And mark where the bleeding ends so that you can see how much time you have to play with before ovulation.

The use of a digital thermometer makes this chore easier for early morning bleary eyes because it flashes the reading on to a little panel. Plot out each day's reading on a special chart. (Booklets of fertility charts can be bought cheaply at chemist shops or at Family Planning Clinics. Or they can be ordered directly from the makers, ZEAL (*see page 62, Chapter 8*).

Ovulation occurs when there is a mid-month drop in temperature followed by a sharp rise to a higher level where the temperature stays roughly the same for the rest of that cycle. The reason for this rise is the increase of the production of the hormone, progesterone, which comes with ovulation (*see page 7, Chapter 1*). Progesterone always makes the temperature rise. This increase also occurs in men if they are given an injection of progesterone for any reason. So the temperature should normally go *up* on the day after ovulation. The higher level of temperature in the menstrual cycle shows that the woman *has* ovulated.

At the end of your cycle, the dots on your chart should be joined up. And do actually join them up with a pen or pencil to make a proper graph, as this makes it easier to see the ovulatory pattern. Do not be surprised if your chart appears different from the perfect printed example in fig. 14 of a smoothish line followed by a precise dip and rise to another recognizable line at a higher level. Yours may go up and down in a bewildering way. But with practice, you should be able to make out the desired pattern.

Temperatures can hop around for all sorts of reasons: a late night, alcohol or illness can send the temperature soaring, whereas an aspirin may lower the body temperature temporarily. Some charts I have seen are initially hard to read. But the difference between the two levels of temperature before and after ovulation is usually discernable and charts become easier to read with practice. Also record on your charts the incidence of personal indications like ovulatory pain or mucus, and see if all these signs coincide with each other. (*See Clare Wright's Chart on page 74 of this chapter.*)

When you have joined up the dots on your graph, you can see the ovulatory pattern that emerges. Ovulation occurs somewhere between the mid-month drop and the higher point to which the temperature rises. *When the temperature drops, start looking out for the slippery vaginal mucus which denotes ovulation.*

When using this temperature method, there is no need to get paranoid over every single reading. If a day is missed, it probably will not matter as long as the ovulatory pattern can be seen clearly. Sometimes, the temperature goes up and down frequently just before ovulation and it is difficult to tell which drop heralds ovulation. When looking back at the end of the cycle, the ovulatory drop will be the one that is followed by a rise to a higher level where the temperature roughly stays for the rest of that cycle before dropping down for the next period. This rise marks the change between the pre- and post-ovulatory temperature levels. Once the temperature has risen to the higher level, you can stop monitoring your ovulatory mucus. It will have come and gone.

By comparing temperature charts over a number of months, see if you can predict the day on which this change in temperature is likely to occur. But I concede that this is a tricky problem to work out before the whole ovulatory pattern can be seen. Recognition of ovulation may have to depend on observation of the appearance of the slippery, ovulatory vaginal mucus (*page 77 of this chapter*).

Take a look at the following examples of different ovulatory patterns. The temperature may rise straight to the high level after the drop. Like this:

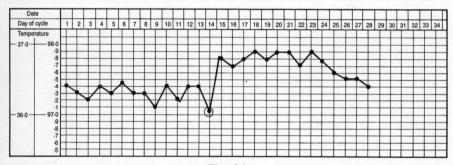

Fig. 14

The temperature may rise in two stages. Ovulation may occur when the temperature drops or when it starts to rise or when it is half-way up, if it rises in stages. Like this:

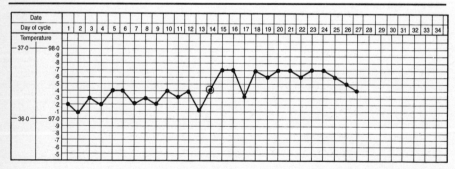

Fig. 15

Ovulation often occurs when the temperature repeats itself. Like this:

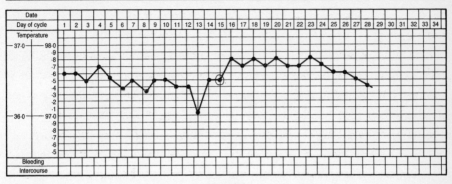

Fig. 16

Clare Wright sent me the excellent chart (on page 74) of her menstrual cycle. It includes all the relevant details and is worth emulating.

- Periods at beginning and end clearly marked.
- Temperature recorded and plots joined up with a line.
- Intercourse recorded every other night up to Day 12.
- Ovulation marked – on Day 16
  - at the mid-month drop in temperature.
  - just before the rise to a higher level of temperature.
  - 13 days before the next period.
- Vaginal mucus recorded and described.
- Personal indications of pains and discharges recorded on specific days.
- Ovulation kit identified.
- LH (Luteinizing Hormone) surge recorded, the day *before* ovulation.

This chart is so easy to read, it makes things look quite simple! Don't worry if your chart looks a mess in comparison. Not many of us can be perfect! But this is the sort of standard for which to aim.

Though even for Clare, ovulation identification is not easy. In her last letter, she wrote: 'My ovulation day is continuing to hop about. You may remember seeing my charts – it varies between Day 13 and Day 21. Last month it was Day 16. We tried for conception five days before but it didn't happen . . . I'll let you know when it does!'

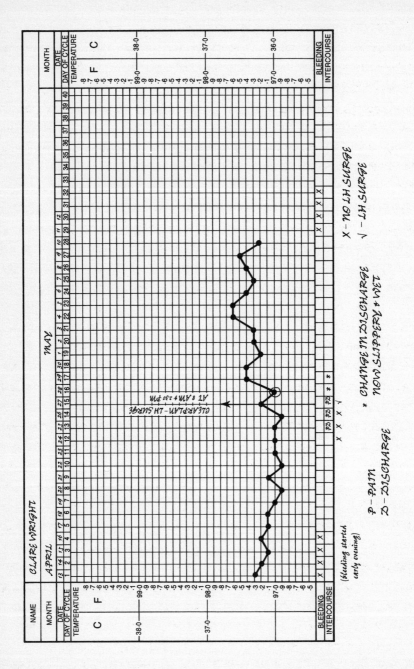

Fig. 17: Clare Wright's Chart

I wrote back that her stopping place should be the first sign of watery discharge which often came as ovulation approached. That was better than waiting for Clearplan which ran things a bit close to ovulation. But there was no harm in using the ovulation kit again, if she wanted a back up. She should keep up the good work and *be patient.* It was hard work to get a girl deliberately!

I wait with confidence to hear shortly of the successful birth of a daughter for Clare, to make up her chosen 'pigeon pair' family. Stop Press! I have just received a phone call announcing the birth of Emma Clare Wright on 4 February 1996. Mother Clare could hardly tell me for laughing!

Personal Indications When making the temperature chart, meditate a bit on what you are doing. Think about how you feel and take note of anything particular you experience regularly, on different days in your cycle, especially as ovulation draws near. Some women report a strange 'feeling' when they ovulate. It is not painful, but they are aware of some bodily function that occurs at the same time in each menstrual cycle. Learning to know the signs of approaching ovulation is called 'Fertility Awareness'.

The most personal sign is found in a woman's feeling of libido which often increases as ovulation gets near. Ovulation is the most fertile time of the menstrual cycle when pregnancy is most likely to occur. Because nature is always interested in furthering the procreation of the species, female animals get a natural urge for sexual relations at this time; they become 'on heat', as it were. However, as intercourse at ovulation produces male offspring, women who notice this phenomenon and want to conceive a girl must be wary, that month, of their natural feelings. They should follow their heads rather than their hearts and have intercourse well *before* ovulation.

Another sign that can be investigated is the changing position of the cervix. This does not stay in precisely the same place throughout the cycle. On non-fertile days, it hangs quite low but, as ovulation approaches, it rises as much as an inch towards the womb. Sensitive fingers inserted into the vagina may be able to feel this. 'A good place to try, is in the bath,' says Tessa Hilton in *Girl or Boy? Your Chance to Choose.*

'Slide a finger into the vagina towards the stomach until you feel a firm lump. This has been described as "a rounded cabinet knob" or "the end of your nose with a small dimple in it". This is the cervix, and you may be able to feel changes in it as ovulation nears and as the os, the canal through to the womb, enlarges and softens. The plug of sticky mucus, impassable to sperm, which usually seals off the os, gives way to the slippery, ovulatory mucus which lets sperm through.' Inspection of this can be another indication of impending ovulation.

Ovulatory Pain About 15 per cent of women experience pain in their lower abdomen around ovulation time. There are two different sorts of pain depending on the time of their occurrence.

Wendy wrote: 'I get a dull ache similar to a period pain which starts a day or two before ovulation and ends when ovulation has taken place.'

Just before ovulation occurs, there is a rush of blood to the follicle which forms a clot and fibre-like tissue. This may be the cause of Wendy's achy pain. This is the German 'Mittelschmerz', the pain that comes in the middle of the month. But realize that *this* pain comes *before* ovulation. To avoid mistakes, a woman has to analyze her pains a bit!

Other women report a sharper pain at the actual moment of ovulation when the egg bursts out of the follicle into the Fallopian tube. It has been described like this: 'A stabbing pain low down to one side which starts strongly and then fades off, leaving me a bit tender.' Or, 'A sharp one-sided pain, like a skewer being pulled through one of my ovaries. More painful than a period pain and lasting over an hour.'

Sue Carter has both sorts:

It starts off mild and bearable for a few hours, then it changes to a very sharp stabbing pain. At this point I have to stay bent over or sitting so that it does not feel so severe. It is like a bad stitch pain and after this the mucus usually shows. Then for the next few hours, the pain gradually eases. This pain lasts for about twelve hours; probably longer if I have already gone to bed with it. Also, I do not get this pain on the same side every month. For two or three months in succession, my right ovary ovulates like this and then a similar length of time follows with the left ovary.

In some women, it is less severe: 'A slight cramp in my abdomen, like wind.' Or, 'A twinge when I ovulate,' and, 'A pain in my back and a lot of raw egg-white mucus.'

Many might regard these women as fortunate beyond measure to have such a notification of ovulation! It certainly helped Sue to get her daughter, Amy, in October 1993.

Vaginal Mucus Most women experience a slight discharge from the vagina at various times in the menstrual cycle. Usually, this discharge is milky, thick and a bit sticky; it is also acid which quickly kills off most male-bearing androsperm. (Do you ever notice a slight staining in your pants at the end of the day?)

At ovulation, there is a noticeable change in this mucus. For a day or two, it becomes wet and slippery, of stretchy consistency like the raw white of egg; this is alkaline in which the androsperm can swim fast. Sometimes this discharge is so slight as to be merely a slippery feeling when you wipe yourself after urinating but sometimes it is more copious. (Do you ever notice a wet lump of translucent jelly in your pants?)

This mucus change indicates ovulation. Make love *once* when you have this mucus, if you want a boy. *Avoid* intercourse when you have this mucus, if you want a girl.

This change in vaginal mucus is the best marker of ovulation. As it is a natural physiological phenomenon, it is more reliable than any man-made gadget. Sometimes, women find it hard to distinguish between the different types of vaginal mucus, especially when these get mixed up with seminal fluid from the last intercourse. But it is worth persevering until you find this reliable sign of ovulation. Look for it in conjunction with temperature taking. When the temperature drops in the middle of the monthly cycle, start looking out for this ovulatory mucus.

A plain wetness or watery mucus often comes on the days leading up to ovulation. This should not be confused with the slippery substance of ovulatory mucus which Jacquie described as 'slime'. This sounds horrible but is really quite a good description!

Women who, for some reason, are on oestrogen medication may be further perplexed because oestrogens stimulate the cervix to produce great quantities of watery mucus.

The changes in vaginal mucus are used by some people as a natural method of family planning. This is known as the Billings Method after the doctor who first described it in 1972. Normally, the tiny canal through the cervix, called the os, is kept closed with a plug of thick mucus which sperms cannot penetrate. But at ovulation, the consistency of this mucus changes to let the sperms through.

By putting a finger into the entrance to the vagina each day, you may be able to learn to distinguish the different types of mucus throughout the cycle, from the dryness early in the cycle to the thick milky acid mucus to the wet pre-ovulatory mucus to the clear, slippery, jelly-like discharge with a stretchy consistency similar to raw egg-white, that comes at ovulation.

For more information about the Billings Method of detecting ovulation send £1 for *The Learner's Guide to The Billings Method* to this address:

The National Association of Ovulation Method Instructors (NAOMI)
47 Heathhurst Road
Sanderstead
Croydon
Surrey CR2 0BB
Tel: 0181 657 1615

Ovulation Kits These kits track the production, in a woman's cycle, of Luteinizing Hormone (LH). Ovulation kits do *not* record ovulation itself, as Yasmin sadly found to her cost (*see page 5, Chapter 1*). They register, in the urine, the surge of LH that takes place just before ovulation, thus giving useful warning of the imminence of this event.

When the dark blue line appears in Clearplan's large window, or when the urine swab in a different kit shows strong colour, start looking out for the slippery ovulatory mucus which is the final indication of ovulation. In some women, ovulation occurs on the same day, soon after the ovulation kit's warning. But other would-be mothers of boys should be ready to wait a further one or two days after the colour change before making love for their son at ovulation. *Wait* for the slippery mucus.

The egg continues to develop after leaving the ovary and Dr Barthakhur in Delhi found that changes in the orientation and positioning of the egg as it was emplaced in the Fallopian tube made it more easily penetrable by the sperm some hours after ovulation. So, there is no need to rush. A few hours' wait or even a day's delay, may be quite beneficial. A good rule is to choose the day when the slippery vaginal mucus is copious.

If there is uncertainty about these ways of determining ovulation, see if they can be synchronized. Does the mid-month temperature drop coincide with the appearance of the ovulatory mucus? And with your ovulatory pain? Do these occur after the ovulation kit shows strong colour?

Try and work like a detective in sleuthing out this prize of ovulation discovery.

Chapter 10

SPERM COUNT IN SEX DETERMINATION

Identifying ovulation obviously must be primarily the woman's responsibility since it is connected with her menstrual cycle.

But we must also take account of the man's contribution to sex determination: his sperm count. The wrong level of sperm count probably has a lot to do with the 18 per cent failure in my results so far. In fact, the success rate of my method has gone up since I started sending out sperm count advice five years ago. There is evidence in this chapter to suggest that sperm count is significant. 'It can even override the timing factor sometimes,' faxed Dr Patel from Delhi. I agree. My research would indicate that:

High sperm count helps to beget a boy.
Low sperm count helps to beget a girl.

During intercourse, the average male ejaculates up to 400 million sperm cells into the vagina. 'Why so many' you may ask, 'since only one is required for fertilization?' Part of the answer is because the vaginal environment is so hostile to sperm. They die off by the million, killed by the acid environment in the complex anatomy of a woman's body. Of those that are left, many lose their way or die of exhaustion.

We saw in Chapter 8 that a high sperm count is required for the begetting of boys because many male-bearing androsperm cannot withstand the adverse conditions they face on their perilous journey through the vagina. Statistically, the more sperm there are, the greater the chance of one of them getting through to fertilize the egg. Hence a high sperm count promotes the begetting of a boy.

Although speed is on the side of the androsperm, endurance is not. Normal androsperm cannot survive long in acid and, if they have been ejaculated into the vagina some days before the egg appears at ovulation, they tend to die off, leaving the field open to the slower but hardier gynesperm.

It is evident that the female-bearing gynesperm have a greater propensity for survival over time than their speedier androsperm brothers, though it is not known precisely how long gynesperm can survive in the woman's body. My own experience, twice, says five days and some of my correspondents claim a female pregnancy after intercourse six days before ovulation. The possible length of the interval between intercourse and ovulation depends partly on the age and fertility of the parents. Twenty-year-old couples are likely to have a higher level of fertility than forty-year-olds, since all bodily metabolism declines with age.

Because of their survival ability, gynesperm numbers do not fall so rapidly, so even a low sperm count has a reasonable chance of fertilizing the egg. Hence a low sperm count can beget girls.

A man's sperm count is very variable and much affected by environmental conditions. Heat is a great hazard for sperm. Sperm count depends partly on temperature conditions in the scrotum, the loose bag of skin containing the testes which manufacture the sperm. The scrotum hangs outside the body, because the testes function best at a few degrees *below* the temperature of the rest of the body. And androsperm in particular develop better under cool conditions.

Thirty years ago in the 1960s, a government report expressed concern at the sudden fall in the number of boys being born. This fact was eventually traced to the current fashion amongst young men for tight jeans which kept the genitals unusually hot. (The Beatles have much to answer for!) Sperm count plummeted, and the result was a drop in the number of conceptions of males. Fashion adverts soon sang the praises of loose trousers and baggy pants.

Although she did not know at first, the heat factor featured prominently in Meriel's life. She had been trying for a long time, some years, to become pregnant but without success. Finally, she became desperate and, with her husband, sought medical advice.

On examining the husband, the doctor noticed a large blood vessel running down the man's groin and delivering a hefty supply of blood to that area which consequently became overheated, leaving half his sperm fast asleep! This reduced his sperm count greatly. The doctor recommended a change of underwear to loose, airy underpants which allowed a cool flow of air to circulate round the testicles thus lowering the scrotal temperature. A heroic twice daily sponging of the genital area in cold water also helped the man to raise his sperm count.

He fathered first a girl and then a boy – after carefully choosing suitable days for intercourse. We can see from this anecdote how a man's sperm count can be altered by environmental conditions.

Some time ago, I received a letter from a young man in Pakistan. Concerned at the wife's inability to get pregnant, the couple had both been for medical tests. She was pronounced fit but Hassan's sperm count was found to be deficient, with 50 per cent of his count dead sperm. He had Oligospermia (Low Sperm Count), with a count of 19 million per milligram, and these sperm were of poor motility. Hassan was distraught. On his behalf, I wrote to Dr John Guillebaud MA, FRCSE, FRCOG, the Medical Director of International Family Planning and Training, in Soho Square, London. He wrote back with very similar advice as that given to Meriel's husband:

Unfortunately, there is really very little that can be done to help any man who has infertile semen; it is an area in which modern medicine is woefully deficient still. The only 'longshot' is to recommend a daily prolonged cold shower in which the testicles are cooled considerably every single morning for at least three months. The reason this can help is because the testicles are outside the body precisely in order to keep them cold. And in some men, if they are cooled even further (especially if the man tends to wear tight pants in a hot climate), there can be an improvement. However, as I say, you have to wait at least seventy days because that is the duration of spermatogenesis.

With this treatment, the sperm would be boosted from their very beginning. Such action would also be a test of heroism! I hope it pays off for Hassan.

Low sperm count has long been associated with female offspring. In Dr Shettles' experiments, a sperm count of less than 20 million per ml of seminal fluid always resulted in the conception of a girl.

This observation shows how futile it is to blame a woman automatically, when a daughter turns up instead of a wanted son. In a sad phone call, Nani, mother of two daughters, told me that she was being persecuted by her family for not producing a son. She had faithfully followed the rules for a boy but to no avail. She was maligned and miserable. Then she persuaded her husband to have a sperm count. This was found to be low at 17.6 million per ml. Hence their daughters.

Knowledge of this fact may have helped to save this family as they know now why they have an all female clan. Their lack of a boy is a sad disappointment, but nobody should be blamed. Nor should there be any aspersions cast on the man's virility which has been proved twice over by the birth of his lovely daughters. Such a regret demands not calumny from the ignorant but sympathy and acceptance from the whole family.

Maybe Nani's husband will try the cold treatment some day? Or maybe they will wisely settle down to enjoy their fine, healthy daughters.

We have seen that in a man with a known or medically diagnosed low sperm count, cold showering or sponging of the genitals is the only accepted method of improving the situation. And sometimes this has surprising results.

With two daughters, Lucy Linolen wrote to me and tried for a boy. She and her husband followed all the rules for a boy but had a third daughter. I suggested her husband have his sperm count taken. This he did through a Marie Stopes Clinic in Manchester and his count was found to be low. Nothing daunted, Paddy embarked on months of cold sponging and raised his sperm count to 46 million per ml. A year later, Lucy rang to say she was pregnant again. Last March, 1994, she produced TWIN SONS! Lucy sent me a big bunch of flowers with a little card saying, 'Thank you, Thank you, Thank you, Thank you!' I marvelled that she had the time!

Cold treatment does not always have such a dramatic effect but it can help in some situations.

Sperm count can be *lowered* in less uncomfortable ways. Heat and frequent sex are the main components of this therapy. No wonder Dr Shettles, the father of four girls and four boys, said, 'Getting girls is more fun!' Though many fraught parents trying for girls might hold that that conclusion is open to debate!

Frequent sex does lower sperm count. 'There is certainly scientific proof of a fall in the sperm count after a lot of sexual activity.' (Hirsh, from *Amelar's First Book on Male Infertility*.) Each time a man ejaculates, his sperm count falls a little. Hence frequent sex is an expedient preliminary in trying for a girl. However, the best interpretation of 'frequent' is every other night; there is no need for the couple to wear themselves out. I have received wry comments from husbands (and wives): What an exhausting time!' The effort demanded is probably exacerbated by the emotional strain.

Stoppard agrees with Hirsh. 'The more often a man ejaculates, the fewer the sperm contained in his ejaculate. It is a good idea (when trying for a boy) to get your partner to abstain from intercourse for a few days so that the number of sperm will rise.' (Stoppard) This is not altogether factual. Abstention does not always *raise* the sperm count (Hirsh). But it keeps the count up to its optimum level. For this reason, intercourse for a boy is best limited to *one* copulation when the sperm count is high.

Dr Hirsh, Andrological Surgeon of Wimpole Street, London, organizes his sperm tests to be carried out after an abstention period of three days as this delay standardizes the tests and makes comparisons more valid.

It would seem that we can further manipulate sperm count a little by noting the words of Dr John Rock of Harvard University, who helped to develop the birth control pill:

Any clothing that prevents the temperature of the scrotum from being at least one degree Centigrade below body temperature, will significantly lower sperm output. Daily wearing of a well-fitting, closely-knit jock-strap *results in infertility in four weeks. Normal fertility returns in three weeks after the removal of the jock-strap.*

A word of warning here. Jock-strap wearing can lower the sperm count drastically. It must be used with care and common sense. To get a girl, you just want to lower the sperm count a little. So, follow these rules:

1 The jock-strap should not be worn for more than *five days*, by day only, in the first month. Reduce this to two days in subsequent months. If still not pregnant after three months' trying, follow Sue's example below.
2 Every *other* night is enough for 'frequent' love-making.
3 If you become very tired and dispirited and your wife does not become pregnant, leave off the jock-strap and just keep to the timing.

When trying for her daughter, Sue wrote that her husband, who had already begotten two sons, lowered his sperm count so enthusiastically that she feared it was now too low to get her pregnant at all. Seven months of intercourse on days exactly right for a girl had not resulted in pregnancy. I suggested that they throw away the jock-strap and wait a month for the sperm count to recover. They complied. And Sue phoned a year later to announce the arrival of their daughter!

(In case my readers do not know, and I didn't know when I was twenty, a jock-strap is a genital support, like a sort of bra, which men wear over their genitals when they do sport of any kind that might be a danger to their anatomy. Jock-straps, small, medium or large, can be bought at sports shops.)

If your man finds it uncomfortable to wear a jock-strap all day (he can take it off at night, by the way), take a tip from Geraldine who got her husband to wear it *over* his pants. He found this method much more satisfactory. And his daughter was born in February 1992, to join her two elder brothers. If hubby still objects to jock-strap wearing, don't precipitate a marital breakdown; close-knit Y-fronts will do as second best!

There are other factors which can lower sperm count. Without doubt, smoking is bad for fertility. Cold sponging or any other fertility treatment would be useless for anyone who smokes eight cigarettes a day. If the smoker gives up, he may see an improvement in his sperm count after three months.

In *Getting Pregnant*, Professor Winston describes one of his case histories: *Richard, a thirty-three-year-old salesman, and his wife, Jean, came to see me after they had failed to have a baby for eleven years. She ovulated rather poorly and had been taking fertility drugs for seven years without a pregnancy. His sperm counts were always low, and artificial insemination had been tried many times without success. We measured his count four times in four successive months. The number of sperm per millilitre varied between 4 million and 9 million, the sperms' motility was never more than 30 per cent and usually about 40 per cent of the sperm showed some microscopic abnormality.*

I advised Richard to lose 20 lb (9 kilograms) and to stop smoking – at that time he was smoking 35-40 cigarettes a day. His work involved driving a great deal, but he didn't feel he could alter this much. I saw him three months later. He had cut down to four cigarettes a day and had lost over 14 lb (6 kilograms). He continued with his normal work but was now exercising twice weekly – for the first time in years. His sperm count on the day of his appointment was 56 million per ml and 50 per cent of the sperm were moving normally, although about 30 per cent still showed some abnormality in shape. His sperm count remained at this level two months later. Five weeks after the second of these two counts, his wife had a positive pregnancy test and, at the time of writing, Jean is in her second pregnancy!

Cutting down on his smoking almost certainly helped raise Richard's sperm count level but steady weight loss was also a significant factor, as was his greater physical fitness. These advantages, combined with his reduction in smoking, soon brought him his long-awaited family.

On the other hand, I recognize that there are some men whose smoking does not have such a drastic effect on their fertility levels. Eighty years ago, my father-in-law was in the Artillery on the French battlefields of the First World War. He smoked often to keep himself sane, and continued when he came home after the war. Nevertheless, when he married twelve years later, he produced a daughter, followed by two sons – one of them my husband (who has never smoked).

But at all events, it is better to be safe than sorry. So, if there is any doubt about sperm count level, I would urge you to eschew the dreaded weed.

Women who want large and healthy babies would do well to join their husbands in giving up tobacco and alcohol when trying for a baby. Both habits increase the risk of miscarriage or underdeveloped babies. And there is a good feeling of solidarity if both partners give up together. Encourage one another!

It is not a good idea to go over the top with excessive exercise and jogging. Physical exercise taken to extremes can also lower sperm count. This will return to normal in six weeks if the exercise is reduced. Moderation in all things!

As we shall see below, alcohol should be strictly curtailed also as, like smoking, it can do terrible things to sperm, affecting motility as well as sperm count. If you want to try for a boy, daily consumption should be limited to three pints of beer, or half a bottle of wine, or 2–3 measures of spirits; the less, the better. If you want a girl, these quantities might help her on her way.

There is as yet no formal scientific proof of a link between sperm count and sex determination. But there is growing evidence, as I outline in this chapter. And, judging from my post-bag, I find constant practical evidence for such a link. Here are some arguments for my belief in the significance of sperm count in sex determination.

1 Many women have written to me bewailing the fact that no matter how carefully they follow the rules about timing intercourse for a boy, they always end up with another daughter. On my recommendation, they have persuaded their husbands to have a sperm count taken and often this turns out to be low.

2 Conversely, there has been an increase in the number of mothers of many sons who have finally conceived their longed-for daughter since I started sending out advice on lowering sperm count. (*See Chapter 8.*)

3 Wives of men who must be away for long (chaste?) stretches, report the conception of a boy on their husband's return, when his sperm has presumably built up to a high level. Our Queen was an example of this situation. Both times when Prince Philip returned after a world tour, his wife conceived another son. (Of course this deduction entails a pretty big assumption!)

4 My observations on the significance of different levels of sperm count are supported by the findings of some reputable medical bodies, especially where the consumption of alcohol is concerned. It is well known that a high intake of alcohol lowers the level of the male hormone testosterone, which is made in the testis and governs the normal working of the testicle in the production of sperm. 'Heavy alcohol consumption in the male can lower sperm count (temporarily) to the point of infertility.' (Health Education Authority [HEA]).

In 1987, a report in the Journal of the Royal College of Physicians* established the harmful affects of alcohol on fertility (high sperm count). 'Alcohol shrivels the testicles and lowers the sperm count by thus reducing the size and efficiency of the testes.' This report showed that men in alcohol-related jobs, who probably drink more than usual, get enlarged breasts and shrunken genitals, and hence a low sperm count. The report also disclosed a lower ratio of males to females in the offspring of such men.

Furthermore, a research team of epidemiologists at the Ninewells Medical School, Dundee investigated this information further and confirmed the findings. Under the leadership of Dr William Lyster, a world expert in child sex ratios, they analyzed the data from the Office of Population Census and Surveys (OPCS) to see if the sex ratio of offspring could be linked to the consumption of alcohol by the father. They found that the ratio of male to female offspring *was* significantly lower in the men whose work was associated with the dispensing of alcohol. For example, restaurateurs and hotel managers, publicans and barmen were 10 per cent more likely to beget daughters than sons.

Moreover, this research group said that other studies they had made

*Journal of the Royal College of Physicians, London. Vol. 21, No. 4, October 1987.

indicated that occupational stresses also altered the sex ratio in a similar way. Here again we can look to the Royal family. The Duke of York is a Navy helicopter pilot, which is a stressful occupation, and he has begotten two daughters in succession. Dr Lyster foretold this and hopes the Duke has seven more daughters to prove the point. I agree with Dr Lyster's deductions but would not encourage such a rash of progeny. That would mitigate against one of my reasons for writing this book – to encourage the curtailment of the world's population.

It is now commonly accepted that stress of any kind can depress sperm production. For some time, I have been viewing with concern the increasing pressures of stress in our society. Many men suffer the despair of unemployment with all that means for the bread-winner of a family. The threat of redundancy, mortgage arrears and the ultimate misery of repossession must be a grinding source of stress. Is it any wonder that, topically (July 1995), the Government is expressing concern at a dramatic fall in sperm count?

The immediate, official reaction was to point the finger at firms like Imperial Chemical Industries (ICI) who produce so many chemical fertilizers that imitate the female hormone, oestrogen. Alkyl-phenolic compounds can mimic oestrogen and cause the development of female characteristics in males. Dr Michael Warhurst, author of the 1995 report, said, 'There is now a huge amount of evidence which shows that many chemicals are able to affect the body's hormonal systems, potentially leading to the reduction in fertility. It is time for action, not more research.' (*Guardian* 25.7.95)

I agree, but I hope such research will not be a red herring to lead us away from the social stresses mentioned above which, I think, may be the real culprit.

OBJECTIONS AND REFUTATIONS

A number of objections have been voiced against my ideas on the importance of sperm count in sex selection. It has been pointed out that there are many other factors which have been shown to shift the ratio of girls and boys born. For example:

1 More daughters are born to older parents.
2 The more children you have, the more likely you are to have girls.

3 First babies are more often boys.

4 More boys are born during the first eighteen months of marriage.

5 During and after war, there is a rise in the number of boys born.

6 A slightly higher percentage of daughters are born to Negroes than to the Caucasian races.

7 The number of girls and boys born changes with the seasons; in the US, June is the peak month for the birth of boys.

8 Some disasters have been followed by a higher female birthrate.

9 Fighter pilots seem to have more girls.

10 Anaesthetists seem to have more girls.

I think all these shifts may be explained by fluctuations in male sperm count, caused by age, abstinence, heat or stress. For instance:

1 It is known that fertility declines with age.

2 Couples who have many children must be fairly active sexually. More sex means lower sperm count means more likelihood of girls.

3&4 Most boys are born to young fathers at the peak of their fertility, soon after their marriage.

5 Men who are away at war have less opportunity for sexual activity. Their sperm count builds up until they have the occasional chance for sex. And when they return home after the war, the hitherto enforced abstention coupled with the lifting of wartime stress may set sperm count at a premium level.

6 I speculate: climate can partially explain this fact perhaps. Negroes came originally from hot climes where warmth is the natural order of the day (and night!). Maybe, they built up a tradition of frequent sex? After all, in many places a hundred years ago, they were denied many other fields of pleasurable activity.

7 Climate again. American boys born in June must have been conceived in September/October when the long, hot summer ended.

8 Disasters cause much stress in most people.

9 Fighter pilots have a stressful job– like helicopter-pilotting Princes.

10 Perhaps working with anaesthetics has a sperm count lowering effect similar to that in the exposure to alcohol (*see page 87, above*).

When these objections are closely looked into, a sperm count explanation can usually be winkled out. It seems that sperm count is a very potent factor that sometimes plays an even more powerful part in sex determination than the timing of ovulation.

In 1979, Dr Roderigo Guerrero of Brazil carried out the most comprehensive investigation to date of sex determination through timing. He studied 1,318 cases and came up with results somewhat in conflict with those in this book. But on reading through his findings again, I realized that he had made the same mistake as I had initially. He did not take into account the importance of the very thing that can override the timing factor: sperm count.

The mean age of the women in Guerrero's survey was twenty-one years. It is likely, therefore, that their husbands were young men in their twenties, at the peak of their fertility with high sperm count. So it is not surprising the Guerrero reports male births resulting from intercourse in the lead up to ovulation (*see page 59, Chapter 8*). As is shown in the table of results on page 91.

CODING OF INFORMATION FOR THE FOLLOWING TABLE

The thermal shift (ovulation) is called Day 0.
Days preceding Day 0 are counted with a minus sign.
Days after Day 0 are counted with a plus sign.

Since, in Guerrero's day, spermatozoa were thought to be incapable of fertilization after three days, Day - 4 was chosen as the first day of insemination by which conception was possible. Day + 2 was considered the last possible day for conception. If more than one insemination had taken place in this period before the shift, the one closest to it was assumed to be responsible for the pregnancy.

At first, I was a bit surprised that the peak day for producing boys in natural insemination was not the day of ovulation itself. But then I realized that, in this survey, intercourse was not restricted in any way and much ejaculation may have taken place during the test week. I speculated that by the time ovulation day was reached, the overall sperm count had fallen considerably. And, as we have seen, low sperm count does not often beget boys (*see page 82*).

Fig. 18: Probability of Male Birth after Insemination in Relation to the Temperature Shift

Day	Natural Insemination Male births	Artificial Insemination Male births
-4	41	9
-3	52	10
-2	61	34
-1	85	67
0	54	100
+1	48	10
+2	23	1

(The figures are large because the sample for this survey was 1,318 couples.)

It is interesting to note that when the doctor recorded the probability of a male birth after artificial insemination (in which presumably the sperm sample was fresh and topped up) the day of ovulation showed a probability of 100.

At all events, sperm count is a factor to be reckoned with. We ignore it at our peril. To have the child of our choice, we must get the timing *and* the sperm count right.

Finally, a letter from a couple who made a mistake and got their much-loved third son, Ben. With further advice from me, they tried again and went over the top in an attempt to subdue what must have been a very high sperm count.

Dear Hazel,

We wrote to you three years ago after the birth of our third son. We had tried unsuccessfully for a girl after reading your book, Girl or Boy? Your Chance to Choose. *We thought we were following your instructions very carefully.*

At this time, we made love only once on Day 10 [mistake], and my wife ovulated on Day 13. The result was not a little girl as hoped, but our 9 lb 2oz boy, Ben. Not that we would be without him now, however. He and his brothers, David (12) and Gary (10), make a great trio.

We wrote to you with our results, and you sent us some more information on the importance of sperm count in sex selection. We did wonder whether or not to try again for our little girl.

After reading your notes and remembering back that with all our sons we never made love any more than once when trying to conceive, we decided to have one last try. [Brave]. We couldn't really work out when Dianne ovulated, as over the last couple of years she has become more and more irregular, with a monthly cycle of anything between 20 and 35 days. But we thought there might be something in the theory of sperm count.

So we set about the exhausting task of making love morning and night for the whole month. With me wearing tight underpants (sometimes two pairs). After a few tiring but enjoyable months, Dianne was once again pregnant.

Then we had the usual first month's wondering, 'Was this the final piece of the jigsaw? Or was Dianne going to be totally outnumbered by males?' At 16 weeks, Dianne opted to have the amnio test done because of her age. She was thirty-eight. She was given the option of knowing the sex of the baby. Dianne said yes, but did not tell anyone she was going for the results.

I was greeted at work by a trembling wife telling me she had something to show me. She then produced a pink outfit she had just bought. Incredibly, the results had shown that she is carrying a GIRL, since confirmed by a 19 week scan and due in February 1996.

We still can't quite believe it has happened. Something my wife has longed for since she was a little girl.

I know some so-called experts may scorn some of your theories, but your ideas on timing and sperm count make a lot of sense. And maybe the sperm count side of it was the important factor for us. Whatever it was, we shall always be eternally grateful to you for giving us the confidence to try one more time.

We're keeping our fingers crossed that the rest of the pregnancy goes well and in February, we'll have our dream come true. Many thanks again. We both hope that you are keeping well and we'll keep you informed of the final result.

Thank you again. Fondest regards,

Terry and Dianne Stamp

I have just received this letter from Terry while his wife is still in hospital:
Just a few lines to let you know that Dianne went into labour on Sunday, and

in the early hours of 12 February 1996, gave birth to our long-awaited daughter, Lucy, and all went very well indeed.

Everybody in the family is very excited as she is the first granddaughter to be born. Lucy now joins the Stamp family ranks, with her three brothers and what a foursome they make!

We can't thank you enough for your ideas, and for giving us the incentive to try again. Lucy was certainly worth the final effort.

Yours gratefully,

Terry Stamp

SUMMARY

ADJUSTING SPERM COUNT FOR SEX DETERMINATION

FOR A GIRL

1 Heat lowers it – tight trousers, warm pants or a jock-strap.
2 Sex lowers it slightly each time – frequent sex at beginning of cycle.

FOR A BOY

1 Coolness can often raise it – loose trousers and underpants. Cold showering or sponging of genitals.
2 Abstention keeps the sperm count level up – intercourse once only at ovulation.

CHAPTER 11

GETTING IT RIGHT –
FOR A GIRL!

'Oh! It's not just for the frilly dresses and ribbons, but for someone for myself. My heart aches for a daughter, a daughter!'

In many countries, the need for at least one girl in the family seems to be more urgent in most women than the need for a boy. 'I can identify with her so much more since she is of the same sex. I know what is going on in her head.' Perhaps this sort of intuitive knowledge is what makes us so catty to other women sometimes! We know how we would feel in the same circumstances, so we can hit where it hurts. But this understanding can also mean an easier empathy and solidarity between mothers and daughters. As we shall see, a daughter is much sought after by most women.

Even in the male-dominated culture of India. 'In the West, as also in the East, any woman will get on more easily and have companionship with her own daughter rather than her daughter-in-law – hence the famous mother-in-law jokes in the West,' said Dr Adi Gazder MBBS, FRCP, DCH, Consultant Paediatrician, Calcutta. He went on, 'I was surprised at the recent increase of childless couples, or with one or two male children, going in for adoption of female children. In India this is especially true amongst the middle class and well-to-do families.' [Where dowries are not so much of a problem?]

As every mother knows, the moment of birth is unique. The physical relief after labour gives way to the all-consuming question, 'Which is it?' Of the bystanders in my day, the mother was always the last to know as she could not easily see what was going on; this always struck me as rather odd! But the question is immediately answered when the baby is put into your arms and you experience an overwhelming flood of emotions. And to find, after only boys, that you have finally produced your chosen girl, is a miracle beyond belief!

'I asked the midwife to go back and check,' said Carolyn Barker. 'Just to make quite sure. I couldn't believe that I had actually borne a daughter!'

'I, Charmaigne Allmans, write to you from my hospital bed to give you the news of our arrival. Are you ready for this? Yes, it's a girl! I cannot believe it! After three sons, we actually have a daughter! There is no word in the dictionary to describe how both of us feel. It worked! The method worked! However can we thank you enough?'

And Nancy Trowbridge wrote:

I felt I had to write in my present state of euphoria and let you know that your timing theory worked for us. We agreed beforehand that it was unfair on the unborn child to hope desperately for a girl and even when my baby was born, I did not ask what sex it was, assuming it was another boy. My husband had said all along that he would like another boy, but his tears of joy when our little girl arrived made us realize that we had achieved what we always longed for.

Love and thanks from us and her two brothers.

I never wanted anything so bad in my life! [burbled Anne Hancock as she recalled the night she gave birth to her daughter, Stephanie, nineteen months after her son, Thomas] *I cannot begin to explain my joy. I was ecstatic!*

After we had Thomas I was shocked by the deep feeling of – not disappointment – but longing for a daughter. I felt so guilty about these feelings and felt I was a very selfish person. Then, I discovered your book and conceived again after four months of temperature taking.

Hazel, I am convinced your method works. You see, I conceived Thomas on Day 13. Because of infertility treatment we timed intercourse for ovulation. I conceived my little girl after intercourse on Day 11. I would like to thank you from the bottom of my heart.

Diane Ashton is convinced about the timing method too.

We didn't use any other method (diet, etc) as what I had read about timing seemed to make good sense. I pin-pointed ovulation on the 14th day and from the third month, we started 'practising'. We followed the advice about getting the sperm count down by regular love-making and keeping the testicles warm. We stopped three days before ovulation and that was it – Hey, presto! Pregnant already.

All the way through the pregnancy, I kept telling myself (and others) that I was not bothered in the least if it was another boy. But, in my heart of hearts, I really wanted a girl. So we were absolutely delighted when, on the 2 September 1993, I gave birth to a beautiful 8lb 8oz baby girl, Zara Dianne.

I cannot say how I would have felt if we had had another boy, but I do know that my face keeps breaking out into a large grin!

I feel sure that following your methods played a very large part in my now having completed my family – for good this time!

Thank you,

Diane and the two boys

There hadn't been a girl born in the Spencer family for six generations. In true tradition, Maria and her husband already had a two-year-old son, Ryan. After studying *Girl or Boy*? very carefully, they decided to 'give it a go!' Maria took her temperature for eight months; she found ovulation very difficult to pin-point but thought it was around Day 14 or 15. In December, they made love freely until Day 11. With no result. Then again in January. With no result. In February, they went up to Day 12 and Maria was pregnant. 'My husband was convinced that it was going to be another boy, but I felt we had given it our best shot,' said Maria. Next October, the 8 lb result was a beautiful baby daughter. The method had worked to complete the family's perfect 'pigeon pair'. Grandpa Spencer could hardly believe it. He welcomed his granddaughter with the words, 'Your parents have broken the Spencer Spell!'

Isabel Audley is equally sure that it was my timing theory that gave her Anne-Marie after three gorgeous sons, Matthew, Daniel and Thomas.

We had always wanted four children and I assumed that with that number, I was bound to get a mixture of boys and girls. It was only after son number three that I began to think about it all. Then I read Hazel's book and the logic of the theory appealed. Getting the timing right would surely tip the balance in favour of a girl just on the basis of the fact that the male-bearing androsperm don't survive as long as the female-bearing gynesperm. I enthusiastically started keeping a temperature chart.

As a former nurse, I had some advantage when it came to reading temperature charts and, after ten months of temperature-taking, I was so expert at studying my cycle I could predict within half a day when I would ovulate. My sons had all been conceived immediately at ovulation but I was so determined to give the theory every chance that I religiously stopped at least two days before my ovulation. For ten months – nothing. And then this harmless, natural theory worked to give us our daughter. Since she arrived she has brought us so much happiness – and it really is undoubtedly thanks to Hazel's method.

I passed the book on to four friends who all had two children of the same sex and it worked for every one of them!

Dr Alisdair Carter and his wife, Yvonne, are unusual in trying the method not once but three or four times with success. They had two sons when they heard of the theory and Yvonne suggested to her husband that they try it, to see if it could bring them a daughter. With typical medical caution, Dr Alisdair demurred at first because the method had not been scientifically proven. Yvonne said, 'Well, I'm going to try it anyway! It's logical and possible.' Alisdair gave in without too much remonstrance. 'It's certainly harmless to try if couples are planning another baby anyway.' He was soon converted by the results, and now suggests it to some of his patients who perhaps want a change this time after having two or more of the same sex.

The Carters got their first daughter, and then another to even up the family. Then Yvonne talked about trying the boy formula for a fifth. In fact, at last count the Carter family numbers six children: 2 boys, 2 girls, 2 boys! I get a photo of them every Christmas and I look forward to the picture of such a handsome, happy family.

But I think now, perhaps, it is time they read the last chapter of the book and called a halt!

Mandy and Tom did the reverse of Dr Carter who suggested it to some of his patients – they were the patients who suggested it to their doctor. After following the method, the doctor had a boy after two daughters.

And I saw something very suspicious at my own local practice in Mill Hill which comprises six doctors, one of whom is Ann. She had three sons. When *Girl or Boy?* was first published, I left a copy at the surgery for the doctors' interest. The next year, I saw parked outside Ann's room, a pram containing a new-born baby girl. Dr Ann was looking very pleased with life. Coincidence? 'Or maybe good timing meant that the last one turned out to be a girl,' laughed the doctor. 'Now, if my patients are keen to produce a particular sex child, I do in fact ask them to contact you for further information.'

As with Dr Carter, husbands are usually a bit more sceptical about the method than are their wives. We have to be very tactful about getting our partners to co-operate; otherwise, love-making to order might lead to the divorce court instead of to the child of our choice. In fact, I am impressed by the devotion and stamina of husbands who nobly comply with the strange requests of wives intent on conceiving a son or a daughter. They co-operate in cold showers or prolonged jock-strap wearing, in marathon stretches of love-making, or being aroused from their slumbers in the middle of the night. Diane Jackson was one such wife:

I would have tried anything. I was very determined. I read in Hazel's letter to me that being hot helps to kill off the boy androsperm. So we only tried for our girl in the middle of the night when my husband had been asleep and warm in bed. And bingo! We got our little girl, Carly, who shines with all our love. It took me one year to fall but she is worth every day (or interrupted night) of it!

Diane's pal, Rita Hart, had three sons. She followed her friend's example 'one hundred per cent' and produced a sister for her boys.

Della Davies wrote after a lengthy effort to right the balance of her all-boy family:

Thank you so much for all your help and guidance over these past few years. I'm thrilled to tell you that we now have a beautiful baby girl, Sophie Louise. Her brothers, all three, are delighted with her. Keep up your good work and advice. We are certain that having sex more often during the first part of the month did the trick. In fact, my husband only the other day, commented with a grin on his face, 'What an exhausting time that was!'

Christine Dorey agrees. The mother of four strapping sons, all conceived after intercourse at ovulation, Christine took her temperature for a year and then timed intercourse carefully. After wearing themselves out with frequent intercourse until two days before ovulation, both she and husband, Dig, were relieved when Christine found she was pregnant. Georgia was duly born and 'sent her mother and all the men of her family over the moon with delight'. Christine is sure that the idea of close-fitting pants helped to lower Dig's sperm count level (obviously high with four sons to his credit!). 'He had always worn loose, baggy pants before.'

The gender balance of the Dorey family has since been further corrected by the arrival of another sister, Augusta.

Veronica Creaney from Essex confirms Christine's thoughts on sperm count:

Our very much wanted daughter arrived on 18 May 1990. Lucy Charlotte is absolutely perfect. I still feel on a 'high'! I can't begin to tell you how much joy she has brought to this all-male family of four super sons. I am convinced that the timing of intercourse in relation to ovulation is the main secret of sex selection. And also, in our case, the lowering of my husband's sperm count played a vital part in our success. I have two friends who tried your method. Both got daughters after already having two sons each. A third friend is on the way and expecting good news soon!

For such fertile parents, it is hard work to get a girl. It is also hard in a different way for women with irregular cycles. But desperate action sometimes pays off!

After a year, Vivien Norton gave up trying to monitor her 'extremely irregular cycles. We just stopped on Day 7 and didn't bother any more about anything. No special diet. Nothing. So the arrival of our little girl was purely down to the timing method. Thank you, thank you, thank you!'

This may have been the rashness of a last ditch stand but Vivien made sure of her girl by keeping to the Day 7 rule even though she had abandoned hope. If 'giving up' helps you to relax and relieves your tension, that is all to the good. As long as you remember the rule, that is enough.

It is harder to get a girl deliberately because it depends on *avoiding* ovulation, and, 'if you don't know when this is coming, what can you do?' puzzled Ruth. Many women, plagued by irregular cycles which sorely tried their enthusiasm for sex selection, coped in various ways.

Alison Farrant had an erratic cycle of between 31 and 38 days. She 'found the consistency of vaginal mucus a better guide. I learnt when to expect ovulation so I could stop in time.'

Kate Young did the same thing by using the Billings Method (*see page 78, Chapter 9*).

Joan Caldwell 'never knew if ovulation was going to be the next day or three or four days away. So, knowing when to stop was a bit of guess work really. But I made temperature charts for six months which helped me to guess right!'

Angie Dallas also, after months of temperature taking, 'bought some ovulation kits (*expensive!*) for more precise results so that we didn't have intercourse too close to ovulation – just in case we got another 3-legged creature!' [I'm sure Angie's humour helped to bring her her daughter!]

As it did with Carys Kinnaird and her husband who 'crept up towards ovulation day by day each month. We made quite a joke of it, so neither of us was uptight. I eventually fell pregnant after intercourse on Day 10, and our icing-on-the-cake daughter was born on 28 January 1990! Thank you for giving us this chance.'

Betty Henry adjusted to a lucky change in her long irregular cycle. After her boys were born, she reverted to a standard 28 day cycle as she used to have before her wedding. 'So instead of waiting, as we had done with the boys, we had sex freely at the beginning and stopped on Day 11. And now we have a little baby girl! Thanks for giving us this chance to choose.'

I take my hat off to these resolute women who succeed with such initiative. My book may have given them the chance they thank me for, but they have seized it with head, heart and assiduous application. They deserve the fruits of all their efforts.

Normally, it is the sexy couples who get rows of girls. They fall into bed and make love as soon as they can after menstruation ceases. And a girl turns up. This laid-back, casual approach should be the recipe for couples trying to get a girl deliberately (*see page 30, Chapter 5*). Make out your timing plan and fix in your head the stopping day. Then, if it is not asking the impossible, forget about little girls! Relax and make love for the joy of it. Girls have a habit of turning up unexpectedly.

After months of temperature-taking, Hilary Turner found she had a long cycle and didn't ovulate until Day 16 or 17. She tried and tried for a girl without success. Ready to give up, she made love up till Day 10 and then got flu.

We stopped everything and I didn't expect anything that month. But I found I was just not getting better from my bout of flu. Then we discovered that my tiredness and sickness were due not to flu but to pregnancy! I did feel bad and hoped that feeling so different from my other pregnancies would mean a change of sex, but I was not convinced until 3 December 1986 when I held my daughter in my arms. I immediately rang my parents at 5 a.m. to tell them!

Influenza also had a hand in the conception of Helen who turned up finally to join her three brothers. Her mother, Priscilla, wrote:

Phil and I had intercourse on Day 9 and Day 11 and then I wanted to try again on Day 12 but he insisted we didn't. I had got fed up waiting to get pregnant, and the number of times we had gone to Day 11 and nothing had happened was really getting to me. Thank goodness, Phil is more patient than me.

Funnily enough, on Day 12 I went down with flu and had to rest for the next few days. My earliest day of ovulation had been Day 14 and the latest Day 21, which is why it took so long for me to get pregnant – nearly a year! I honestly feel that because I was not thinking about whether I was going to ovulate on this day or that day, and because of the rest I had to have because of the flu, meant I got pregnant. I also had a high temperature, so whether this helped just the female sperm to survive I don't know. Anyway, I do know that Helen survived it! I still find it hard to believe that I have a little girl. She is lovely and is adored by all the males in the household!

If you want to use my name and address for people trying to have a girl, don't hesitate to put me down. I remember how I needed to write to other people who had tried. So once again thanks for all your help. Every time I rang you, you were always very supportive. I really appreciated that and the fact that you never made me feel a nuisance. You were the only person who never made me feel guilty about wanting to know ways of influencing the sex of your child. Lots of other people must be feeling like that – wanting to know but not knowing who to ask or where to get information. Please write again if you need to know anything else at all.

From me, my husband Phil, Carl, Adam, Luke and Holly, bye.

P.S. I lost my own mother when I was seven years old so it is nice to have a mother and daughter relationship again.

Lucinda Talk's daughter came as a surprise too.

My second son was barely nine months old when I saw Hazel's book in a shop at Epsom in Surrey. I immediately bought a copy and rushed home to start reading it. I couldn't think about anything else! I took my temperature every morning for twenty-one months but found my charts very different to the examples in the book. With this in mind, we decided to give it a try, though, to be honest, we didn't think it would work.

We just casually made love for the first five days after my period and then did nothing for the rest of the month. I thought we had made love in my 'safe' period and I didn't expect anything that month. I was amazed when I did a *test and found I was pregnant! On 19 October 1988, I remember clearly my husband proclaiming, 'We have got what we wanted!'*

I cannot begin to describe what I felt. Rachel was here as we had chosen! My parents are besotted with her and she is the first girl in my husband's family for two generations! Without your book, I am fairly certain we would not have had our darling daughter. She has made such a difference to this family which I now feel is complete. To have a mixed sex family is so lucky because each sex has something to offer and can give so much pleasure. And I think my tear-away boys have become gentler since their sister arrived. Thank you so much.

P.S. I have kept all my charts and dates of ovulation. If you ever need such information for future research or articles, I would be only too happy to help you.

The comment of Lucinda's on the effect of a baby girl on her elder brothers is echoed in many other cases. When asked for their opinion before the birth, young boys are often definite in their preference for a brother who can be macho with them.

'No mamby-pamby girls for us! If you bring a female into this house, we shall kill it!' So my nephew Gordon, and his wife Dee, were told by sons David (4) and Matthew (2), when they ventured the hope of a coming baby girl. But when Elizabeth arrived, the boys became 'strangely fond and protective of their little sister'. Sororicide has not been mentioned again. Dee says 'Elizabeth's coming has transformed my life. I never feel sad or lonely when she is around.'

Jackie Lloyd's sons of six and three 'protested at first and said they wanted a brother' but when Katie came male hearts were touched. The three-year-old crept in to gaze in wonderment. 'Can I touch her? Oh, Mum, isn't she beautiful!'

But the frilly-pink-dress stuff sometimes doesn't last all that long. The three he-men brothers in Kate Tutty's family saved their men-only club by making their sister into an 'honorary' boy! And, when I went to visit the Wilcox family in Cumbria, I couldn't, at first, pick the girl out of the five boys who rushed down the hill to greet me. All with cropped hair, in shorts and trainers, they looked like a regular football team! Nevertheless, 'Chloe rounded off our family perfectly!', her mother had announced with relish five years earlier. Tomboy or beauty, she was a *girl*!

Yady Stroud wrote:

The difference she has made to our family is phenomenal. We all feel so happy and proud of each other; and so clever! In addition to my joy in having a girl, I now feel even prouder of the boys because now I can appreciate the difference; that they are not just our children but boys and girls! Lydia completes our family perfectly. She was a granddaughter after four grandsons – a real fairy-tale story but absolutely true!

Often, the extended family, especially the grandparents, join in the celebrations with heartfelt joy. 'My mother was dumbstruck at the news,' said Pauline Davies. 'She had waited twenty years for a granddaughter! I spent most of that day crying with happiness.'

For some lucky mothers, the whole choice palaver is a complete fairy-tale:

Our daughter, Jessica Lauren, is perfect! She was delivered at home on the day the hospital computer gave me. My waters broke, and she was born. It was all just perfect! We have a beautiful daughter to prove your method works.

Yours most truly grateful. So happy,

John and Jane Fisher
James, Daniel, Benjamin and Jessica

Anne Holloway had no trouble either:

We already had three boys and decided to even up our family. With three children, we found that one was often left out. If the fourth were to be a girl, it would be a bonus.

I took my temperature for three months and found it very easy to pin-point ovulation. As well as the timing, I kept to the girl diet in Hazel's book. But once I had ovulated (and possibly conceived?) I returned to a balanced diet – to make sure my baby was getting the best. I had a girl! I was delighted and so were the boys – mainly because they didn't like the name I had chosen for a boy. (Aren't children grand!)

Denise Baxter calmly followed the rules exactly to get her two children.

For the birth of our son, we had intercourse on the day of ovulation, Day 14, and for our daughter, we tried four days before anticipated ovulation. As we are both in our thirties, we are delighted to have achieved the family we wanted at the time we wanted. I hope this letter encourages other couples to plan their families as successfully.

However, some mothers have a long traumatic struggle.

Clare Andrews first wrote to me in November 1991. The mother of two sons, she was desperate for a daughter. She had been hunting for months for her ovulation day but her charts showed a different day each cycle – Day 14, Day 19, Day 16, Day 13. I suggested she watch her vaginal mucus to determine ovulation and reckon the days by her shortest cycle.

5 December 1991 Clare was pregnant! Temperature chart showed intercourse up to two days before ovulation – right for a girl.

10 December 1991 Miscarriage. 'I just feel destroyed,' cried Clare.

19 June 1992 Five months' pregnant but on a very erratic chart with frequent drops and rises. Which drop marked ovulation? How does she know? Feels OK.

12 October 1992 Third son born!

14 January 1994 'I have been trying every month up to Day 9 for the last ten months. I am on chart 10 but I can't make head or tail of it. My youngest is 15 months now, and he is just wonderful – an absolute bundle of fun as are his brothers. I love them all dearly but a little girl would still be just perfect. What do you suggest?'
I replied:

What patience and persistence! What energy! I suggest going up to Day 10; Day 9 was obviously too early to stop. Perhaps you are trying too hard for a girl which has maybe given you a psychological blockage against pregnancy (see page 30, Chapter 5). Stop thinking about it so much. Just casually make love up till Day 10, thinking about each other, instead of little girls. I hope you get pregnant before you both have nervous breakdowns! Love-making must seem like a bit of a chore. Don't let it be. Buy a new nightie and return to romanticism. Then your daughter may surprise you!

30 September 1994 'Well, I've finally done it! I've got my daughter! And I haven't really slept since I had her as I still can't believe I've got a girl. My husband, Richard, and I are over the moon – still floating on cloud nine. The boys, Ashley, Perry and Jesse are thrilled to bits with their sister. Her nickname for the moment is Sunnie, because she has brought a ray of sunshine into all of our lives. But her real name is Ruby, which brings constant flashes of delight. I feel I am going to burst with the love and pride I feel for my wonderful family. I am so really happy I sometimes cry as I can't believe it has all worked out so well, thanks to you and your book.'

So it took Clare four years of effort and heartbreak to get her daughter. It is a harsh fact that all too often a miscarriage occurs when a woman finally conceives a baby of the opposite sex from the one she had before. But Clare had the guts to try again, and eventually her body co-operated.

With two lovely sons of eight and six, Keith and Pauline Loven tried again and again for a girl. Twice Pauline got pregnant and twice she miscarried after severe sickness. Then she stopped ovulating for a year – due to stress, she thought.

I was ready to give up but your letter was very encouraging, so we bravely decided to try again. We made love early in the cycle and waited. I wasn't sure that I would ovulate at all, as I hadn't for months. But things progressed as normal and I was delighted to find myself pregnant. Again, I felt extremely sick for the first twelve weeks but there were no complications, and our long-awaited daughter was born! She was baptized at Easter. I enclose a picture of our elder son, Alex, cuddling his baby sister, Katherine Elizabeth. Many thanks for our beautiful girl. She is an absolute delight!

It took Helen Porter six years and two sons to get her daughter. This was not because of illness or miscarriage but because she made a mistake in counting the days of her cycle. She was confused about when to start counting. She got two or three days of 'spotting' before her period started properly, and she didn't start counting until the real flow began. That was her mistake. The cycle begins with the first sign of bleeding even if it is only sparse brown smudges of blood. That is Day 1.

This mistake explained the conception of Helen's sons when she thought she was trying for a daughter. When she reckoned she was three days before ovulation, she was in fact precisely there. If her calculations had added on the three days of spotting at the beginning of the cycle, she would have realized that their love-making hit the day of ovulation exactly. No wonder they had boys! Five years and myriad letters finally cleared up this misconception and in 1991 I received another letter:

Having written to you several times during the past six years, I am delighted to be sending you this announcement of our daughter's birth! We made two mistakes in miscalculating Day 1 of my cycle which brought us our lovely sons. This time – five days ahead – we were successful and the icing is finally on our cake! Laura was born in September and the feeling is worth a million pounds!

With our thanks and best wishes,

Mike, Helen, Daniel, Alexander and Laura.

Sara Windsor and Susan Ash agree. 'If it weren't for the method in your book, we probably would never have had our lovely daughters. Now we are content and happy. Words cannot express our gratitude.'

'Women tend to extend their families until they obtain the sex they strive for, though many would not admit it.' So observed Kate Hall as she persuaded her sceptical husband to try the method for a sister for their son. 'To my husband's amazement and my joy, it worked and I gave birth to a little girl. Now I feel fulfilled and happy.'

'With two strapping sons', Richard and Christopher, Gaynor Weatherley tried and tried for a daughter and got her beloved son, Adam, instead. Gaynor described her cycle as 'completely haywire', and she sent a large bunch of temperature charts from 1992 on, for me to decipher. This was hard! We eventually decided to reckon on Day 15 as a likely ovulation day. Intercourse was stopped on Day 12, but Gaynor was uncertain as to the precise day on which she ovulated. Could I predict her chances for a girl this time?

Below is a copy of Gaynor's last chart. What would *you* have said?

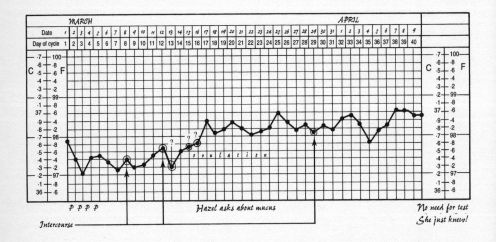

Fig. 19: Gaynor's Last Chart

I wrote back:

> If you ovulated with the temperature drop on Day 13, that would probably be too close to the intercourse on Day 12 for a fertile couple like you to get rid of all the androsperm before ovulation. So another boy would be likely. If however, as I think, you didn't ovulate until Day 16, just before the sharp rise to the higher temperature level, that would be just right for a girl. Only you can tell by observing your vaginal mucus and noticing when it was slippery. When was it?

On 6 December 1995, I found out when I received this announcement:

> I did it at long last!

> Gaynor, Paul and Boys are very pleased to announce
> The arrival of a girl!
> Katie Louise   wt. 8lbs 6oz
> born 6.12.95   time 8.40 a.m.
> at
> Barratt Maternity Home, N'pton.
> I'm still floating on a cloud – will write in the New Year.

The other side of the world can show us how it is done! Here are letters which say it all:

> Dear Mrs Phillips   Queensland, Australia

> I enjoyed reading your book, Girl or Boy? Before I bought your book, I had already given birth to five boys, four of them planned on the day of ovulation and one accident. I'm sure that happened on the day of ovulation too!

> I love my five boys but longed for a daughter, my own little girl. Friends and family all had a mixture. Why couldn't I? You know the old saying: 'A son is a son till he gets him a wife. A daughter's a daughter all of her life.'

> I'd heard about the theory of timing and decided to try. We wanted a large family anyway. I bought your book and proceeded to pin-point my ovulation, mainly by mucus observation and position of my cervix. My husband and I had sex freely until three days before ovulation. (I was a textbook case exactly, with ovulation on Day 14, fourteen days before my next period.) I conceived straight away but unfortunately miscarried at eighteen weeks. It was a girl. I was very upset, but consoled a little with the fact that a girl was possible. We waited three months and then tried again. Nine months later, my daughter,

Lauren, was born! We were all very happy. My sons had hoped for a sister. Lauren has brought joy into our family and the desperate longing in me has gone.

I only wanted six children really, but I would like to try again for a little sister for Lauren. Five boys and two girls sounds good, but if I should have a little boy I wouldn't be disappointed, because the desperation is gone. To be real honest, when my daughter was two days old, I actually felt a little sad. As I was so used to little boys, I kind of missed him. Funny, isn't it?

I believe there is a lot of peer pressure to have a certain sex. When my fifth son was born, I was proudly showing him off to an acquaintance when she said, 'Ah, poor you! How unlucky can you be?'

I hope this letter has been of some help.

Yours sincerely,
Anne Nikolic

P.S. THANK YOU!

Auckland,
New Zealand

Dear Hazel,

I wrote to you in the latter half of 1986 enquiring about your sex selection method. I had received from the National Women's Hospital here in Auckland a letter which totally contradicted your sex selection theory.

After receiving your reply I was confused as to which theory was right. I took your advice and purchased a copy of your book, Girl or Boy? from Thorsons.

I had my copper IUD removed and waited three months before trying your method. In the meantime, I started taking my temperature in the morning; this was always erratic. But I always have a 28 day cycle and I noticed I had a jelly-like discharge from the vagina on the fourteenth day of the cycle. I found this more reliable than taking my temperature.

As we already had two sons, James and Jared, I wanted a daughter. My husband had no particular preference but was willing to try out your theory.

We took your advice to reduce my husband's sperm count by having intercourse twice a day. The first month, we had sex up till three days before ovulation. I did not conceive, so the next month we went up till two days before ovulation. And I conceived, much to my husband's relief as he was pretty worn out!

For the next three months, I was violently ill and lost one and a half stone in weight. I went to my doctor who gave me acupuncture to ease the constant vomiting. That made me feel a lot better and I was pleased not to be hospitalized. I had had vomiting when pregnant with the boys but not as severe. My doctor jokingly suggested I was carrying a baby of the opposite sex!

The rest of the pregnancy went smoothly and on 5 September 1987 I gave birth to a beautiful 4 kg daughter, Laurel!

My husband was ecstatic and my sons were thrilled to have a little sister. Since her birth my eldest son, who was always a bit aggressive, has become more gentle-natured. Laurel is five months old now and I constantly relive her birth over and over in my mind. The thrill of having a daughter after two lovely boys has made me a complete person. We only wanted to have three children and I know, if I had had another son, I would have felt that something was missing in my life. Don't get me wrong. I would have loved the baby dearly whatever the sex and I am grateful that my children are healthy and happy, which is what is most important.

I am sure your theory is correct and I have a queue of friends waiting to borrow the book. I am very interested to see what results they have. I would like to say thank you for writing the book and putting forward your theory which was easy to follow, and natural. I hope my letter has helped you with your survey of results.

Yours faithfully, Diane Cathcart

Finally, this chapter draws to a close with the contentment of two loving mothers with four sons apiece – and a daughter!

Margaret Wilcox from Cumbria, purchased *Girl or Boy? Your Chance to Choose* while staying with relations in Bristol.

We had four boys and didn't really intend to increase our family. But after reading the book, the method appeared so absolutely logical that it seemed worth a try. It was easy to avoid the middle of the month as I always had a slight pain when I ovulated. And my husband was away all week at University, so I knew exactly when our daughter was conceived – after intercourse well before ovulation.

What a difference Chloe has made to our family! The boys are so proud of her! She's very special. What more can I say? I can still hardly believe it! The village school was delighted, but our parents were most put out when we announced a further pregnancy; 'people don't have big families nowadays'. However, when their first granddaughter was born, things were quite different! Friends and neighbours were so jubilant for us; we received over 100 cards. One local lady said, 'God rewards a trier!'

What actually inspired me to write was a postcard from a doctor friend who read your book and has just given birth to a daughter after two sons. Not only her, but two other friends who already had two sons, have produced daughters after using your method. It really does work, and I have no hesitation in recommending your book to everyone.

I am so glad I read the book after my fourth son; otherwise we might not have had the last three, and that would be unimaginable! Thanks for the method. We are complete now,

Margaret

Both previously married, Steve and Gina Watts had three sons between them. After their wedding, a fourth son came along to join his brothers. As the product of their new union, Daniel was very precious. But he was another boy, and both parents longed for a daughter. The book *Girl or Boy?* gave them hope. Gina felt that, as the boys grew older, they would be doing more and more activities that didn't include their mum. With a daughter, she could share so much.

The parents followed the rules exactly and in three months, Gina was pregnant. She felt very smug and convinced that she was carrying a girl. The pregnancy felt quite different from her previous ones.

Then the Clinic told me that it was a large baby, bigger than my sons had been, and I suddenly thought it must be another boy. I felt very down about it. But, after a while I picked myself up and put all thoughts of having a girl out of my mind. After a long and tiring labour from Tuesday morning until Wednesday afternoon, I delivered – a large, lovely daughter! She was so beautiful, none of the midwives said a word. They left it to my husband to tell me. We were ecstatic, both crying tears of joy. Her brothers absolutely adore her. They all wanted a sister; they had 'got enough brothers'!

Her full name is Lauren Jade. Jade because, like the precious stone, she is very precious to all of us. She has made us utterly complete. Perhaps the happiness we feel every day is thanks enough, Hazel.

With love,
Steve and Gina Watts & Co.

This chapter ends with the glad news of the arrival of a girl after two boys. This is the commonest situation in my post-bag. And it takes much courage to risk another child in the hopes of a daughter. Congratulations to those who dare – and succeed!

Dear Hazel,

I bought your book when my husband and I were deciding to have another baby.

We already had two boys and I thought it would be nice if we could do something more positive about trying for a girl, although we wanted another baby whatever sex it would be.

I will try to answer your questions in the following text.

We used the temperature method to pin-point ovulation when we were trying for our first baby (not having been told by the doctors that once ovulation has occurred the chances of the baby being a boy were high) but we did not mind what sex it was.

Our second son was conceived in a most 'natural' way, i.e. we weren't using contraception and it just happened on holiday.

I had always had a regular menstrual cycle so it was easy for me to pin-point ovulation when we decided to have our third child.

I read your book and changed my diet in favour of a girl, used the temperature method again and specifically the timing before ovulation for conception, and this is what I believe to be the key in determining the sex.

I know exactly (to the day) when my baby was conceived. I went all the way through my pregnancy thinking it would probably be a boy (not wanting to build my hopes up too much). My midwife even said she thought it was a boy (from listening to the heartbeat) so you can imagine my absolute surprise and amazement when my daughter was born! I was so completely surprised it took me a few days to get over the shock. I couldn't believe how lucky I was that I had actually had a girl and it had all been worth it.

I felt a little bit guilty about the fact that if it had been a boy, would I have been so elated? Probably not, but I think it was the shock that surprised me so much.

I feel 'complete' now we have a mixed family and can indulge myself with pretty clothes for her.

So thank you from the bottom of my heart, for giving me the information I needed to conceive at the right time.

If we decide to have any more children, I feel equipped to make another choice — though next time it won't be quite so important and after all a baby is a joy and a gift from God, whatever the gender.

Yours sincerely.

Mrs Amanda Moore

CHAPTER 12

GETTING IT RIGHT – FOR A BOY!

As you have read, there have been lots of families with only boys who wanted, and got, a daughter. According to my records, the families who had only girls and were keen to have a son, were less than half in number. A possible explanation for this may be:

- Ovulation is the most fertile time of the menstrual cycle.
- Many couples know this and, when they plan a baby, head straight for intercourse at ovulation time.
- Normally, boys are conceived when intercourse takes place at ovulation.

Therefore, boys are conceived more readily than girls, when a first baby is planned.

It seems to me that, on the whole, it is the calculating couples who usually have sons first after their union because they make sure they have intercourse at ovulation time. Nature, always keen to ensure the survival of the species, encourages this behaviour by increasing a woman's libido as ovulation approaches, so that her sexual interest in her mate grows as she nears the moment most favourable to conception. If you want a girl, you must resist your instinctive feelings at ovulation! The more naive (like me and my husband in our youth) just make love with gay abandon from the beginning of the menstrual month. And we find ourselves with a row of daughters!

In 1986, I got a letter from Janet Pocock, alias Jenny Jones, who was *miserable*. Aged forty-two, she had four daughters: three in their twenties and the youngest aged fourteen. All healthy, all bonny but all *girls*. Janet was so desperate for a boy. Every day she schemed and plotted how to get her dream. She wrote to medical men in London, went to see them and wept on the doctors' shoulders. She felt time was running out. She was galled. Then she found my book! *Girl or Boy? Your Chance to Choose* gave her one last chance.

Because of her age and because her husband would not think of another baby, Janet decided she must arrange for her son by herself and in secret from her husband. As she had only one ovary, she planned carefully for two years. She changed her eating habits to the book's boy diet, she bought (and hid) temperature charts, she used Discretest Test Ovulation Kit, she wasted £50 on gadgets that she couldn't get to work. She tried anything and everything. She was obsessed. To maintain the secrecy, she called herself 'Jenny Jones' and used a friend's address for me to reply to.

I had to do it in secret [wrote 'Jenny'] because my husband wouldn't have agreed. I told him I was using the calendar method of contraception and he swallowed it hook, line and sinker. I only agreed to make love when my mid-month temperature dropped on Day 13 [exactly wrong for contraception!]. Every month I fobbed him off with a 'headache' or something until that day. It was the Devil's own job to get him interested on the day! I used a bicarb. douche before intercourse and timed my orgasm to precede his. Everything went to plan perfectly and I became pregnant. After three months, I had a scan. I asked them, 'Can I buy things in blue?' They said, 'Yes!' I nearly fainted with happiness. I was delirious, yet scared I would miscarry. Happily, I didn't.

On 3 March 1988, Oh Joyous News, as they say!

I HAD A BOY! Normal at 10½lbs!

What a shock for his dad who idolizes him completely – and for his sisters!

I confessed my plot to my husband after the birth, and now he laughingly tells everyone how he was tricked into it! But he doesn't mind; he's got a son now. He carries him everywhere, and the pride just glows on his face! Words cannot describe our feelings. We've got a son, Hazel, and it's all down to you! Nobody thought it was possible. Even after four months, I can't believe it. We call him Thomas Toby. He's beautiful and we worship him! Thank you for giving me a chance to select a son. Thanks!

Love from,

Mrs Janet Pocock and Baby Boy, Tommy

What a letter! I chuckle every time I read it! Although I don't recommend this type of marital deception, however brave and single-minded. Obviously, Janet was very close to her husband and knew that he could take a joke of this kind. But of course, ideally, children should be wanted and planned by both parents in conjugal love and concord. Janet admits that, on looking back, she doesn't know how she had the nerve to do what she did. Supposing she had got a fifth daughter? She thought she would have killed herself. But having said that, she remembered how much she loved her daughters even before their brother came along. And his miraculous arrival has doubled the mutual love of his family for each other.

Debby and Adrian Barnes also got their son at their first carefully planned attempt.

I was shopping in Boots one day and your book caught my eye, so I decided to buy it and try. We had two lovely daughters and were thinking about a third child. If we could improve our odds for a boy, we were ready to give it a go. I read your book eagerly from cover to cover. Then I began doing my temperature chart faithfully for two months. We decided that the third month would be goal. After my second period, we started the diet theory as well. I improvized the potassium suggestion for a boy by eating a banana a day. Somewhere in the back of my mind, I recalled that bananas were high in potassium. [Correct.] I also made my husband do the diet – it certainly would improve our odds.

Well, as C-day (Conception day) approached, my mucus was there and my temperature was up to 98.2 F that morning, so we knew tonight was the night. We had abstained from intercourse for the week before and we followed the 'missionary style' position. [Really the position for a girl!] We made sure I had an orgasm first, and it was just a one shot try.

We then crossed our fingers (and I my legs for a bit) and waited to see. Nature took its course and within a few weeks I knew I was pregnant. The doctor soon confirmed it. Time passed and my bump soon became very active. When my contractions eventually began, the midwife counted the heartbeat and reckoned it was a girl. (Now, I had been hearing this for two months – but in my heart I felt certain it was our son.) Well, finally the head came peeping up at us and then the little one's body. My husband shrieked, 'It's got two umbilical cords!' The midwife advised him in no uncertain terms that that was a boy!! The tears began to flow and my whopping 9lb 4oz son had made us the two happiest parents in the world! – for the moment.

*Now the sleepless nights dominate our minds and we are certain that boys
are much more demanding than little girls ever were! However, we still feel
very fulfilled and send our grateful thanks to you, Hazel.*

These two cases support the theory that it is easier to try for a boy because it just
means accurately pin-pointing ovulation instead of trying to forecast when it is
likely to happen. But careful temperature-taking and fertility awareness is still
needed, as Viv Austin found out. She had heard that ovulation takes place on the
fourteenth day and that boys were more likely to be conceived then. She
followed this plan for her next child who turned out to be an adorable second
daughter.

'Then I read about Hazel's method and sent for her book,' says Viv. 'When I
followed her advice and started charting my temperature, I soon noticed that I
didn't ovulate until Day 16.' Viv made sure she conceived her third baby after
intercourse at ovulation on the sixteenth day and the result, nine months later,
was the chosen brother for Lauren and Emma.

Carole McCarthy is also firmly convinced that it was timing that gave her and
her husband their son, after daughters Chelcie and Sophie.

*I was very interested in your easy and natural theory as to how to get a son. I
followed your instructions completely and on 1 March 1993 I gave birth to
Harry. My copy of your book is now permanently out on loan! Many thanks
for all your help. Both sexes of children have much to offer and I am so glad to
have had the chance of both.*

Carole

It may be an irrational vestige of past days, but it seems that many women,
myself included, feel inadequate or a failure, if they have not given their husband
a son.

*I knew my husband wanted a son very much [wrote Carole Feltwell] because
he was the last of the line and wanted to continue his family name. If I didn't
have a son, I would know that my husband was disappointed and I would
probably feel that I had failed him and must try again.*

*Then we read your book. My husband is a trained scientist and helped in
understanding the principles involved and in making sure the temperature
was taken accurately. Our son, Thomas, was born this year!*

*Our four year old daughter is delighted with her brother and, for myself, I
am very relieved that the pressure (albeit very subtle pressure) is off me. I feel*

that to have provided my husband with the son he wanted has made me 'a success'! We are both very happy.

We feel that your book enabled us to consider the whole matter of the conception of our children in a much more controlled way and we are glad that we were able to use the method to our satisfaction. Several of my friends are now reading the book!

Roslyn Feeney felt 'incomplete and lacking something until my son bowed in to join his two sisters who were conceived after intercourse early in my cycle.'

Grace Pilditch, 'was a little sad at not having had a son. Having James after reading your book has made a fantastic difference to my life. He makes me complete, somehow. Though I love all my children equally – I have no favourites!'

Gillian Paul suspects, 'I would have felt I had missed out on something, if I had not had a son as well as my lovely girls.' Gillian had irregular cycles of 30–32 days.

So we decided to work backwards. The first month, we abstained until Day 18 (my longest cycle minus 14). I didn't get pregnant. The second month, we abstained until Day 17. I was pregnant and our son was born in the autumn, exactly two years after reading your book! He is a joy! A perfect 'monster', and we shall always be grateful to you, Hazel. When people ask me 'How did you manage a boy the third time?' I recommend the book!

I purchased your book two years ago [wrote Susan Stevenson]. At the time I had three beautiful daughters aged six, four, and two, and it's hard to put into words how I longed for a son. I kept a special place in my heart just in case one came along.

For six months I charted my temperature, using a fertility thermometer. I found this fairly easy to take and read and each month I noticed the sudden rise at ovulation time. All this time I made sure I wouldn't get pregnant until I had learned the pattern of my cycle. Then we tried for our son. We abstained from love-making until the day of ovulation and didn't have sex again that month until after my period was due. It was unbelievable how quickly I fell pregnant on that day. In my previous attempts to get pregnant with each of the girls, when we made love freely before ovulation, it took about six months each time. My husband and I just couldn't believe I'd conceived first time like that.

And to make things even better, the baby was due in 1990. We'd always wanted a baby in that year!

Sure enough, on 12 January Christopher James Stevenson was born! That was two weeks ago now, and my husband's eyes still fill up every time he holds him. He thought the method silly at first, but now you have a non-believer turned in to a true-believer. Our lives seem very fulfilled now and our three daughters love their little brother as much as we do. Thank you,

The Stevenson Family

Leslie Kanaah was not so successful at first. Having two daughters, she hoped for a son. She

bought a kit on ovulation (£20) which turns urine blue when ovulation occurs. [No! This is a mistake heading you for disaster! (See Yasmin on page 5, Chapter 1).] *Making love at the blueness, I was pregnant by November and soon found I was carrying twins! Twin boys? That would be lovely. After a wonderful, carefree pregnancy, out popped twin girls! I was delighted and relieved that everything had gone so well. But I knew, even though he tried to hide it, that my husband was disappointed. And everyone else made things worse. As soon as I rang to tell them, relations, friends, etc. all said, 'Oh, really? Are you disappointed?' This really upset me, as twins are such a precious gift as I'm sure you would agree.*

Anyway, the main reason I am writing, as well as sharing our experience on the outcome of this situation, is this. We have coped so well and both adore our four girls but we are seriously thinking, at the end of the year, to try one last time for a boy. I have timed my cycle for the past four months which has shown 27 days, 28 days, 26 days, 28 days.

So when should I try for a son?

I wrote back, congratulating Leslie on her lovely children and giving her the same advice as I had given to Yasmin. Two years later, Leslie wrote again.

I finally gave birth to our little boy, making our family complete. Our little girls love him! Thanks Hazel, for the information you sent us.

The Kanaah Clan

Leslie's story shows how critical it is to hit on precisely the right day. Chemical changes in the body happen so quickly that it is imperative to identify accurately the day of ovulation. Merely counting days and 'hoping for the best' will not do, as Susan Lea found to the cost of three charming daughters.

I married at nineteen and wanted a family straight away. We started as soon as my period finished, and the next April my daughter Claire was born. We tried once more a couple of years later, straight after my period again and daughter, Sarah, was born.

I was a little disappointed to have another daughter. The whole pregnancy and birth were so different from the first; I was quite surprised to be told, 'A little girl.' I've always loved little boys and wanted a son of my own. I was fifteen when my brother, Nigel, was born and I adored him and used to pretend he was mine.

We had planned a family of three so I hoped it would be third-time lucky. We waited for seven years; in that time I had read various press and magazine reports about timing and ovulation. I came to the conclusion that I had had two daughters because of having intercourse early in my cycle. [Clever girl!]

So we waited and abstained from sex until my fourteenth day – I have always been lucky with a 28 day cycle, so I knew I could pin-point my days just by counting. [Not so clever!]

We conceived the first month and in June 1983, my big, bouncing third daughter, Rebecca, arrived. I was very surprised although, after a seven year gap, not as disappointed as I expected to be. We decided we were destined to have daughters only and that was it.

Over the next couple of years, although I adored my daughters, it was constantly on my mind of wanting a son. We were sure it must be something to do with ovulation and that Rebecca just missed being a boy. In 1985, I bought your book.

So in August 1986, we decided to try just once more. This time we knowingly waited until Day 16/17. In July 1987, my son, Jamie Peter, was born a healthy 9lb!

My whole family were ecstatic! And we are thrilled with our happy and contented son.

Susan Lea

Harminder Jaspal also found the value of learning exactly how her body worked.

Initially, I used to find the temperature plotting a little confusing. However, eventually I became more aware of my body and its discharge, finding the mucus changing with a dip in the cycle. It is with the greatest of pleasure I am able to write to you that I actually gave birth to a little boy on 23 March 1993, after following your rules exactly.

Many thanks from myself and my husband and daughters. We found your personal communication and confidence inspiring; which gave us that push. And now we have a perfect family of three lovely, healthy children of both sexes.

Your sincerely,
Harminder

The logic of the method appealed to Rita Gleason as it had done to Nurse Isabel Audley (*see page 96, Chapter 11*).

I knew that my two daughters were conceived after intercourse straight after a period so, after reading your book, it made a lot of sense that the opposite was for a boy.

I asked my husband to read it but, I suppose, like a lot of men he was a bit sceptical and apprehensive. He didn't believe in sex selection; 'thought the law of averages had a lot to do with it.' But he was very patient and said he would go along with anything I said, as he was desperate for a son as much as I was.

I found your method so easy to follow. I didn't bother too much with the diet – just went off milk and ate lots of salt and chocolate. Hazel, my husband really believes in your book now. We still cannot believe we have a son! He must have known how much he was wanted as he is a very happy baby and as good as gold. We are thrilled with our son and so are his two sisters. He has brought us so much happiness; our family is complete now.

Rita Gleason

P.S. I first read about your book on the problem page of Woman's Own and I sent for it straight away. Thank you for it; it's a wonderful book!
P.P.S. While pregnant, I was 80 per cent sure it was a boy as I had timed it to perfection.

Some women find it harder work to time things so accurately. Mrs Mutti told that:

I first tried on Day 16 but failed to get pregnant. Then you told us to try Day 17. The next month, we missed the date and tried on Day 18 and that failed too. Then we tried on Day 17 which was Christmas Eve. I missed my period and yes, I was pregnant! After that, all was well and in September, I had a beautiful baby boy. Thank you a million times over! We've done it! We've got a lovely boy after two beautiful girls. Thank you for looking at my charts and taking time to talk to me on the phone. Once again, thanks a million!

I think this sort of personal contact is helpful. When you write a book and put your ideas into print, you lose immediate control of their message. I tried to write clearly in *Girl or Boy?* but obviously failed in some instances. I knew exactly what I meant to say but, to my regret, my readers sometimes misunderstood crucial points. (*See Linda, page 53, Chapter 7*). This is why personal communication with me or with somebody else who has successfully tried the method is valuable whenever possible. By exchanging addresses, I can often link together mothers who are going through the sometimes lengthy trauma of trying to get a girl or boy deliberately. It can be comforting to compare notes and sympathize. We are starting quite a Choice Syndicate!

Gynaecologist at two London hospitals, Yehudi Gordon, MB, Ch.B, MD, FRCOG, agrees: 'Thank you for all the help you have given over the years to the many people that I have referred to you. With one exception, they have got what they wanted.'

Over the past thirty years, 98 per cent of the couples I have seen personally, in face to face consultation, have been successful in getting the child of their choice. I can answer individual questions and make sure that the method is fully understood. Of course, not everyone can come to see me, but the phone does well as second best.

Forty-one-year-old Sarah Kingham had two bonny daughters of twelve and ten. Sarah had been trying in vain for five years to learn the trick of getting a son. Her doctor did not see her problem. She went to her local fertility Clinic and complained that she could not get pregnant with her long irregular cycle. The Clinic put her on Clomid which regularized her cycle. Then Sarah found my book.

Phone calls flew back and forth from Northampton to London until one afternoon in December 1990. Sarah rang me to say that she was experiencing the slippery, vaginal discharge which she thought must denote ovulation and what should she do? I suggested immediate bed and one round of love-making. Mr and Mrs Kingham complied that night and Sarah became pregnant. Nine months later, Sarah delivered a healthy boy to join his delighted sisters.

You will notice that Sarah was put on Clomid to regularize her cycle and she had a son.

Many women have written to me worried that they will not be able to conceive a son because their doctor has put them on to Clomid. It is true that this drug often seems to encourage the conception of a girl, and I think the following may be the reason.

Oestrogens are the hormones which develop secondary female character-istics. The drug, Clomid, occupies oestrogen receptor sites in the hypothalamus, thus interfering with the feedback mechanism. This means that more oestrogen is produced, giving rise to the theory that females will ensue. But, in practice, the intercourse-at-ovulation-for-a-boy rule can often override the extra amount of oestrogen and the birth will be as usual, a boy – or even two!

Joanne and Stephen Cherry were teachers and as such were very used to chart-making! Just as well, since they were under the doctor's care for fertility treatment. Joanne was not ovulating properly and was put on to Clomid. Their GP 'kept a close eye on them' and encouraged them to try for pregnancy at ovulation. This they did twice and, as standard, got two sons! Then, naturally, Joanne longed for a daughter.

I had become quite expert at reading my fertility charts and looking for the mid-month drop. With a willing husband, I kept creeping nearer to the magic 14th Day, but staying before it. After six months of trying, I eventually managed to conceive after stopping on Day 12. The absolute bonus of a result – Judith Alexandra Ruth – arrived on 7 October 1988! I didn't really believe the doctor and mid-wife when they said, 'It's a girl!' I asked them to let me see and check for myself! Undoubtedly, your guidance helped us to achieve this precious gift and we are very thankful for your help,

Stephen, Joanna, Stewart, Chris and Judith

However, before her girl, Joanne had had two boys while she was on Clomid.

Here, a word of warning from Professor Winston for those on Clomid. Because this drug increases the number of follicles and therefore the number of granulosa cells in the ovary (*see page 5, Chapter 1*) the progesterone level *may* increase to a misleading level, even though you have not ovulated. If you don't fall pregnant within three months, check with your doctor that you are ovulating properly.

Unlike Joanne who couldn't believe the outcome, Vivienne Piccini was more like me and 'knew immediately' that she had conceived a son. And 'the completely different experience of this pregnancy confirmed my conviction that I was carrying a boy. Baby Barry joined his two sisters to complete our family perfectly! I hope my experience has been of interest to you and I'll be passing on your method to anyone interested.'

Sue Tragenza noted the mid-month drop and rise in her temperature and got the timing exactly right for the son she had planned as a brother for her four-year-old daughter. But sadly, after three months, she had a miscarriage (*see page 105, Chapter 11*). Sue spent a few months mourning and regaining her peace of mind. Then she tried again at the temperature drop. Nine months later, she was 'over the moon' after the arrival of David James. Her husband hasn't stopped showing him off and Grandpa joined his daughter on cloud nine when he welcomed his first grandson. David was very special as Grandpa and Grandma had had only daughters themselves.

Abroad now. In August 1988, I received a frantic phone call from Heathrow Airport. Bruna Floris had picked up my book to read on the flight back to Italy. She phoned me at the last minute to get more information.

Well, I didn't try in August but waited till September so I could follow all your instructions. Thank you so much for your help because I succeeded and now here is a wonderful boy who is six months old. I'm enclosing some of his photos herewith. Doesn't he look beautiful and happy. My husband and I are jumping out of our skin with joy. It is a real miracle! I can't express my gratitude for all your help and encouragement. I do wish you all the best for your life and a Merry Christmas and a Happy New Year!

Then this letter came from Madrid.

We are very pleased to tell you about our experience of having a baby pursuant to your method of choice of the sex of the baby. We would like to inform you of our previous history.

We are a couple that have been married for two years; previously we got married with other people. From the former marriage, we have three daughters, one from my wife and two from my side. So we decided to have a new baby, but we strongly preferred to have a boy than a girl, and started to read some books about the choice of sex. We bought your book at the end and got very interested in it due to the high rate of success in comparison with other methods.

It was not easy. At first we tried for several months and nothing happened. We were very upset because we thought we were not able to have a baby of ours. So we decided to visit a doctor, who made us several tests: sperm tests, vaginal liquids test, and everything was fine. So he told us that since we were completely compatible we had only to wait and not get nervous. Eventually we had a boy as we strongly wished.

After our history I am going to tell you how we did it.

We already had three daughters before our present son.

We carried on the graphic of basal temperature for several months to find out the ovulation day.

We knew exactly the ovulation day with the help of our doctor who told us the most likeable day in relation with the graphic.

We were sure of the moment of conception because I was on a trip and back home that day. At night we made the intercourse.

My wife carried on a diet but not very strictly at the same time and we managed to get the boy we hoped. Our son is the only boy and the only one in the family, so all of us are very happy.

Thanks for your help and I apologize for my not good english.

Senores De Quero

Now to the other side of the world.

Just as Scottish Clans used to need a Laird to support them, so Indonesians in Sumatran Suku need a male Penghulu to direct the affairs of the family group.

Wahidar Anwar of West Sumatera is an old friend of mine. For seven years we had brought up our families near each other in Mill Hill while both our husbands taught at London University's School of Oriental and African Studies (SOAS). The trouble in the Anwar family was the fact that no boy had been born for seventy years. Wahidar had followed her family's usual pattern and had given birth to three beautiful daughters. But she was determined that one of her daughters should provide the missing Penghulu.

In 1982, the Anwar family returned to Sumatera. Soon the two elder girls were married and, in true family tradition, produced a daughter each. Wahidar found an excuse to visit me again and procure three books which she handed round to her daughters on her return to Indonesia. (Wahidar felt that she had given her daughters a chance to get a son by themselves but now, perhaps the gentle push of my book was required!)

The eldest daughter, Dewi, finished her Ph.D. at an Australian University, returned to Indonesia and put Hazel's book into practice. Pregnant again, Dewi and her husband, Yos, felt in their bones it was a boy. They were very shaken when a scan predicted another daughter. However, six months later, they were doubly thrilled when it was a boy after all! The first boy in the family since 1920, Deka's birth was quite an event! He is all set to be their Penghulu in later life. And now the second daughter, Danti with husband, Anton, has followed her sister's example and had a boy too! Fortunes have certainly turned around in the Anwar family. And Dewi has 'told quite a few interested mothers about the method'.

Another good friend of mine is Nitaya, a Thai woman married to an Indonesian, Oking Gandamihardja. With two pretty daughters, Tasha and Tania, born within a year of each other, this family also lived for some years in Mill Hill while Oking worked for SOAS and the Overseas Service of the BBC.

One day, when Nitaya and I were hunting through Nitaya's diary for some particular date, I noticed a Thai word which kept recurring at regular intervals throughout the diary. I asked what it was and Nitaya told me it was the Thai word for ovulation. She was keeping a private record of her cycle, safe in a language which not many people in Britain understood! A year later, her son, Yuri, was born!

Ani Santiko was a mature student at SOAS. She was taking an M.Sc. in Archaeology and she lodged with us for a year. She and I chatted about everything under the sun, including babies! Ani had two daughters aged nine and six whom she had left at home along with twenty-seven pet cats! After finishing her research at the University over here, Ani picked up a copy of *Girl or Boy? Your Chance to Choose* and left for Jakarta. A year later, I heard that Ani's thesis had been set aside temporarily in favour of more pressing interests. Ani had had a son and was 'over the moon' as she described it. This expression is constantly used by many happy mothers.

It seems that super-lunar space must have become overcrowded recently.

And the moon rises in many parts of the world.

From Pakistan, Maryam Bashi wrote to say that, with God's help, the recipe for a boy had worked for her to produce, after five daughters, a son!

From Nigeria, 'The book is doing a wonderful service to humanity,' wrote Jonathan Olubi, the proud father of a son after five daughters. Jonathan's doctor friends are trying the method on their patients because 'a mixed family is best so that both fathers and mothers are represented. Bravo to you, and much grease to your elbows!'

And from the wide open spaces in Australia where they still enjoy large families, came this crisp letter.

Dear Hazel

My wife and I recently decided to have another child and we read your book, GIRL OR BOY? Thank you for the assistance you gave us.

We already had three children and all were girls.

We thought it would be good to try for a boy.

We were able to pin-point ovulation through the Billings Method.

We feel sure we knew when the baby was conceived.

The only method we tried was your own.

We did get the boy we hoped for; in fact, we got two boys: 200 per cent success rate.

Your book was easy to read so thank you for your help.

Warwick Chesters

Here is a letter that says everything, from Sonya Kennedy of the Baulkam Hills, NSW. Failure is followed by success!

Dear Hazel

Our little boy is nine days old already and I still can't stop smiling. It only seems like yesterday that I wrote to you telling you about the miscalculated birth of our third beautiful baby girl, Jade, who is now twenty months old.

I received your letter with sperm count information, after Jade was born and, as we had always planned on having four children, we started charting my cycles as soon as I started menstruating again. (About six months after the birth.) They were fairly regular even though I was breast-feeding for twelve months.

We decided to go to a Billings teacher and were taught that method until I was positive of my ovulation time. I discovered through charting that I actually ovulate on the third day of my ovulation pain, not on the first day like I initially thought. (See page 78, Chapter 9) I had reckoned on the first day when Jade was conceived, so in fact I was sure to have had a third girl because, with Jade, we had intercourse two days prior to ovulation. So, in fact, she proved your method to be correct 100 per cent. We also read Dr Shettles' book and followed your further advice on Hugh wearing boxer shorts for a couple of months prior to conceiving. This time we conceived first attempt and I felt positive now that my calculation of ovulation was spot on.

On 12 March, 9.10 a.m. I gave birth to a beautiful, healthy boy, Aaron, weighing 7lbs 15 oz. We were thrilled! Jasmin, Amber and Jade just adore him. And what a lucky little boy to have three older sisters! We have now got just what we always wanted: four children – three girls and a boy. I can't believe it!

As you can imagine, we are quite busy but absolutely loving every minute of it. Hugh loves helping; it is great to have a husband who is really involved in the family. It is something really special.

Hazel, thanks again for sharing your knowledge through your book.

Fondest regards, Sonya

What determination! What persistence! I am amazed at the doggedness of women in pursuit of a son! When you realize that any mistake means a commitment for life to a child you did not choose, the risk becomes daunting. Nevertheless, the desire for children of both sexes drives women to take this risk.

Professor Winston disagrees with all the antics we women get up to. He treats it all as a bit of a joke, saying of acid douches, 'My feeling is that your vinegar would be better employed on a green salad!' I have my suspicions that most doctors would say these strange procedures put too much stress on a couple's love-life. That may be the male doctors' viewpoint. But I maintain that the letters in this book show that women (and often husbands, too) willingly put themselves under such stress, if it means an end to the helpless acceptance of whatever their undirected bodies produce.

Writing about infertility, Professor Winston says, 'I have found that if a man and a woman can find the reason for their infertility, it is very much easier to come to terms with the distress it causes.' I think this is true of any disease, and also of the initial disappointment which follows the arrival of a child of unchosen sex. A great deal of stress is lifted when such parents understand why their child was conceived. And more stress evaporates when they feel they can do something to swing the balance to the sex they choose. And even if, for some reason, women get it wrong, usually their maternal instinct bravely accepts the new life in motherly love. Jo cuddled her third son and said, 'It is better to have tried and failed than not to have tried at all.'

The Greeks and Romans were not the only ancient peoples who have had ideas on sex selection (*see page 35, Chapter 6*). Early Jewish writing and tradition had some interesting theories which still succeed in producing boys. And they fit in with my theory very well! There is something in Jewish Law that has a significant bearing on sex selection. A spokesman for the Jewish Board of Deputies in London told me that research into this question had been carried out in Israel, and this research did indeed show a greater proportion than usual of male births among Orthodox Jews in Israel. I wondered why.

At an Open University summer school, I was discussing sex determination with another student, Evelyn, who was the Jewish mother of a mixed family. She said to me in a matter-of-fact way, 'Of course, I waited till the day of ovulation to get my son.' I was curious again, and asked her how she knew.

Evelyn told me that when she was a little girl, she had sat at the knees of her grandmother who was a religious woman and who used to read the Talmud out loud to her every day. (The Talmud is a compilation of Jewish laws and customs dating from the 4th century AD.) This reading became like a sort of folk-lore to Evelyn who assimilated the precepts unconsciously so that when she reached womanhood she followed naturally in the traditional rites of cleanliness as stated in the Talmud.

Fascinated, I delved into the Old Testament and ran off to the library to study the sixty-two volumes of the Talmud. And this is what I found concerning Jewish laws of cleanliness after menstruation:

If a woman have an issue, and the issue in her flesh be blood, she shall be put apart seven days; and whosoever toucheth her shall be unclean until the even. (Leviticus 15 v 19)

For the Orthodox Jew, the Talmud goes on to say this:
Subsequently however, it was enacted that she must wait seven days from the end of menstruation. (Pesahim, Vol. 2, p.579)

Now, with the usual menstrual cycle of 28 days, this ruling would bring the woman right to the day of ovulation. Moreover, she would have abstained from sexual intercourse from the beginning of her last period.

I began to wonder less at the Jewish tendency to have boys! I have many Jewish friends and they nearly all have at least one son.

I went on reading the Talmud and found this:

If a woman emits her semen (has orgasm) first, she bears a male child; if the man emits his semen first, she bears a female child. (Tohoroth: Niddah, p. 217)

It seems that the theories put forward in this book are nothing new. The Jews have been practising them for centuries! But sometimes, they find it difficult to beget girls!

A preponderance of boys was evident in this letter I received from Sandra (Feldman) who had married into a Jewish family.

Dear Hazel,

Last year I wrote to you for advice after purchasing your book Girl or Boy? Your Chance to Choose, *as there has not been a girl born in my husband's family for sixty-two years. My husband is one of four brothers and the two brothers that have married have two or three boys each so it was no surprise when my son was born last year. But I was keen to have a girl somewhere along the line.*

You wrote me a lovely letter back. [I had asked if she was by any chance Jewish, as that might explain the dearth of girls in her family. Sandra confirmed that her husband was a strict Jew.] *And after following your rules, baby Laura arrived on the 28 October 1983, weighing 8 lbs 1/2 oz.*

As you can imagine, we are absolutely delighted and I want to thank you for writing the book and for your subsequent advice. I recommended this method to a work colleague who also produced a girl earlier this year. Thank you once again.

Sandra Feldman

Ten years ago, my doorbell rang to reveal a young woman with a pretty, dark-haired, little girl. Mrs Rhoda Levy was on her way home after seeing her GP about having another baby. 'I want a boy this time, Doctor. How do I go about it?'

Doctor Allan told her he wasn't in the business of sex selection but said, 'Go up to Mill Hill and see Hazel Phillips. She knows a thing or two on this subject.'

So, Rhoda came in, and I asked her:

'Are you Jewish?

'Yes.'

'A strict Jew?'

'Yes.'

'How come you have a daughter then?'

Rhoda smiled sheepishly. 'Oh well, things don't always happen as ordered, do they? It was a hot, romantic night . . .'

I smiled back and told Rhoda how to get her boy. Two months later, she reported on what she had done, keeping strictly to the Jewish Law and I said, 'Congratulations! I think you are carrying your son. When he is born, take him and show Dr Allan the proof of the pudding!'

This she did with alacrity, when her son arrived.

So, my method is not just a presentation of what people have been doing privately for a long time. Some need to be alerted to the rules – though others may suss out the maxim for themselves.

Maria, an old woman from Cyprus, wrote approving the book, 'You are quite right, you know. I have been telling this method to my villagers for years.'

Some years ago, I was on a BBC chat show for Radio Wiltshire and Mr Fred Morris (68) from Trowbridge, told me how he and his wife had used the method twenty-four years ago. 'It was printed in some magazine, I forget which.' [I have such an article in an old copy of *Woman's Own*.] 'We used it to get our son, eleven years after our three daughters. We were sure of him as soon as he was conceived. Nine months later, when I rang the nursing home, Tilbury, here, to find out the news, the matron said, "Oh, Mr Morris, she has delivered . . ." I interrupted, "Oh, yes, it's a boy isn't it?" Matron couldn't believe that I knew!'

Many people have got their mixed families by working things out for themselves. My cousin, Susan Driver, who trained as a nurse thirty years ago, married John and had a daughter, Lucy. Three years later, her son Alistair came along. When I asked her how she had managed it, she said simply, 'Well, of course, I waited for ovulation to get my son.' Did nursing training help perhaps?

This rule holds for most people who happen to make love on ovulation day. And for those who do not bother to work things out, there is often an unexpected turn of events.

Mothers may write books and propose, but children dispose in their own way – congratulations to my own first-born, Sheena, and her husband, Chris!

My son-in-law has just phoned from Edinburgh with the happy news that his son is safely born – in the bath! Like many second-born babies, Matthew Richard shot into the world unexpectedly quickly to join his brother, Jamie, nine months after a romantic Easter holiday, when his parents had recklessly followed their natural feelings of love without a thought for the timing rule (*see page 66, Chapter 9*). And this bundle of fun was as heartily welcomed as was his brother before him. As the Scots say, they make a bonny wee pair!

In March 1984, I joined in some correspondence in the *Guardian* on sex determination. David Amess MP had voiced worries that the practice of sex selection would upset the balance of the sexes that we currently have. I hastened to reassure him with the following letter.

After 30 years' research into a highly successful method of natural sex selection, I hasten to reassure David Amess MP and other fearful parties that the long term practice of sex selection will probably lead to a more accurate balance of the sexes than at present.

In the thousands of letters I have received from enquirers all over the world, only one request was for a child of the same sex as had been previously born to the family concerned.

This desire was for reasons of economic convenience: the family house had only two bedrooms and the parents wanted to put their two girls in together.

Apart from this case, all women in my experience want the sex they have not yet got. Mothers of girls want a boy; mothers of boys want a girl. Most want a small family; many are satisfied with one of each sex.

Mothers do not envisage raising armies, nor do they wish to upset the balance of the sexes. But they do wish to experience the full potential of motherhood in bearing and rearing children of both sexes.

The desire in women to choose the sex of their children is the most natural wish in the world and nobody should be ashamed of it.

On the arrival of the other sex, most mothers write echoing the words of Gillian Clark: 'Thank you. We are complete now.'

What interested me in the *Guardian* the next day, was the letter from Christopher Hay, a GP in Bromsgrove, Worcs., that followed mine. Such a witty summary of my method delighted my eyes. Here was a perfect example of someone who had worked it out for himself. Of course, Dr Christopher Hay had the advantage of medical training. But his 100 per cent success is certainly better than that of the Gender Clinic!

Anybody can alter the odds of which sex child they conceive – without needing all the paraphernalia or expense of the London Gender Clinic.

Boy sperms are more fragile than girl ones (a bit like when they're grown up, some would say), and won't last as long if they don't get the chance to fertilize an ovum within a few hours. So what you need to do for a boy is maximize the chances for their vulnerable sperm – and try to conceive immediately after ovulation. For girls it's much easier to kill off the male sperm by stopping sex a couple of days before ovulation is due – it'll be a bit frustrating and make conception a bit less likely each month, but put the odds in favour of a girl.

Of course, small numbers don't mean much when you are just tinkering with probabilities – but we've had a hundred per cent success rate so far (boy, girl, boy), which is better than the figures that we've heard of from the recent press reports (four out of six – 67 per cent). And thankfully, we've got nobody to blame but ourselves if we get it wrong.

Christopher Hay.

Bromsgrove, Worcs.

And here is another valid viewpoint.

I am one of three daughters. I have no brothers. The media is suddenly rendering my family 'incomplete'. It is absolutely ludicrous.

Nan Gruffydd Jones.

Cardiff.

CHAPTER 13

DIET IN SEX DETERMINATION

I'll start by being frank. I hate diets of any kind! Usually, they are a pain for the dieter, a pain for the cook and a pain for the rest of the family. However, I realize that some unfortunates need a diet for medical reasons and they have to suffer this burden.

Diet figures large in people's thinking these days. The right diet is promoted as the cure to many problems. I know many people with multiple sclerosis who happily torture themselves with unpalatable foods in the hope of a cure. And some of them swear to an improvement in their condition as a result of their diet. Unfortunately, the recommended MS diets forbid all the things I love. So it became of great importance to me that I find an argument to reason away the diet! I was helped in this by an article written in the *MS News* by an eminent specialist in the disease. He suggested we made a list of all the diets supposed to help MS. Then we should scrump it up and throw it in the waste paper basket, as MS is not cured by any diet. I hastened to do what he suggested!

This course of action was corroborated for me by a nurse from the National Hospital for Neurology at Queen Square in London, which is situated near London University's School of Oriental and African Studies where my husband works. When staff from SOAS go abroad to Asian countries, they need to be inoculated against tropical diseases, and nurses from the National Hospital are often employed to do this. My husband, Nigel, chatted to the nurse while she gave him his injections:

'In your job, you must know about MS. What can I do about my wife who eats all the wrong foods and loves chocolate and cream?'

'Oh dear! Does it make her very fat?'

'No, it doesn't seem to do that. She has always been pretty slim. She doesn't eat very much of anything – except chocolate.'

'Well, forget it then. She may as well enjoy it, if it doesn't make her fat. She must have a fast metabolism. She is lucky!'

I say amen to that, and have another chocolate!

I am not suggesting that all MS patients should eat chocolate. Only the lucky ones! If you are on a diet which helps you, stick to it and congratulations on your resolve! I am just explaining that I eschew diets of any kind.

I have always been dubious about the diet method in sex selection because I found it unnecessary. I did not change my diet before conceiving either sex of child. In fact, my natural preference was heavily weighted towards the dairy diet recommended for conceiving girls. Maybe that explains the early arrival of my two daughters? I think not; as I did not change my eating habits when I tried for and got my son. I only changed the timing of intercourse.

The French Dr François Papa admits that it is a long and gruelling task to change the body's chemical make up through diet but he claims to do it as a means of determining the sex of offspring. On the other hand, I think that the natural secretions of a woman's body at various times in the menstrual cycle are more significant. Get the timing right and your hormones will do the rest for you in providing the relevant mucus. Nature's sex selection does not work by so clumsy a method as diet change. So what is this chemical change and how can diet help? Let us turn to France. Trust the French to find the answer in food!

Dr Papa is consultant gynaecologist at the Port Royale Hospital in Paris. He worked out a diet theory for sex selection based on four vital mineral salts found in the body. These are:

1 For boys: Sodium and Potassium (powerful alkalis based on alkali metals)
2 For girls: Calcium and Magnesium (from Carboniferous limestone rocks)

Sodium and Potassium attract male-bearing androsperm (y). Calcium and Magnesium attract female-bearing gynesperm (X). The clever idea of the diet is to alter the chemical composition of the egg so that it attracts the desired sperm.

FOOD TO GET A BOY

As much salt as possible: salted butter, salted and smoked meats.

All meats, fresh or pre-cooked. Especially beef, since cattle are often treated before slaughter, with male growth hormone, which is then passed on to the consumers of the beef. Of course, this is rather dubious in the light of the current BSE threat. Other meats may have to suffice.

All fish, and two eggs weekly.

White bread and white-flour crisp bread.

White-flour cakes, pastries and biscuits.

Pasta, rice, semolina (all without milk).

Milk-free puddings and sauces.

Most vegetables (except those forbidden below): sweetcorn, popcorn, parsley, mushrooms, courgettes, endive, avocado, fennel, raw tomatoes, soya beans, peas and beans, chestnuts.

All fresh fruit, particularly Potassium-rich bananas and fresh pineapple.

Dried prunes, raisins, figs, apricots.

Sugar, jam, fruit jellies, sorbets.

Oils and milk-free margarines.

Soups, olives and gherkins.

FORBIDDEN WHILE TRYING FOR A BOY

Milk in any form – butter, cheese, yoghurt.

Shellfish, molluscs (mussels etc.).

Wholemeal bread.

Salad vegetables: raw cabbage and cauliflower, spinach, cress.

Nuts, cocoa, chocolate, mustard.

FOOD TO GET A GIRL

As much milk as possible ($1\frac{1}{3}$ pints or 770 ml per day).

Fresh cream, yoghurt.

Limited meat or fish ($1\frac{1}{4}$ oz or 125 g per day).

Unsalted butter, unsalted soft cheese.

Milk puddings.

Salt-free wholemeal bread, crisp-bread and pastry, without yeast.

Rice, pasta, semolina, tapioca.

Limited amount of potatoes.

Fresh or frozen carrots, green beans, turnips, aubergines, onions, leeks, peas.

Cucumber, radishes, peppers, cress, celeriac, celery.

Unsalted walnuts, hazelnuts, almonds, peanuts.

Fresh, frozen or tinned apples, pears, clementines, strawberries, raspberries.

Tinned only pineapples, plums and peaches, all *without* syrup.

Jam once daily, sugar, honey.

Vegetable oils, spices, home-made sauces without salt.

Mineral water.

FORBIDDEN WHILE TRYING FOR A GIRL

Salt and salt substitute. All salted or smoked foods, including salty cheese.

Coffee, tea, tinned fruit juice, fizzy drinks.

Wine, beer, cider, liqueurs, aperitifs.

All meat and fish, except for daily allowance above.

White bread, pasties and biscuits, unless salt-free; crisps.

Sweetcorn, popcorn, parsley, spinach, cabbage, cauliflower, mushrooms, courgettes, endive, avocados, fennel, raw tomatoes, soya beans, dried peas and beans.

All fresh fruit except those listed above as allowed; dried fruit.

Chocolates and sweets.

Bicarbonate of soda and all prepared sauces.

All ready-made dishes whether tinned, fresh or frozen.

Now a word of *caution*. If you suffer from certain conditions, *these diets may be dangerous for you*. The salty, boy diet should *not* be undertaken by anyone who has high blood pressure. The girl diet should *not* be undertaken by anyone who has kidney stones or high blood calcium levels. If in doubt, check with your GP first.

And make sure that any restrictions you put on yourself don't lead to an unbalanced diet. A plentiful supply of nutritious food is essential just now to you and your unborn baby. When all is said and done, the health of parents and baby is of paramount importance. If the diet upsets you in any way, come off it. Dawn Osborne said her cycles had become unpredictably longer since she had been following Mr Hewitt's diet. And the high doses of Vitamin C gave her diarrhoea and made her feel ill. So she stopped. Nevertheless, Dawn and Darren got their daughter by sticking to the correct rules for timing and sperm count. Kristina joins her big brothers, Matthew and James.

But, if you really want to try a rigid diet, contact:

Mr Jonathan Hewitt, MB, Ch.B, MRCOG
Consultant Gynaecologist
Liverpool Women's Hospital
Crown Street
Liverpool L8 7SS
Tel: 0151 708 9988

Mr Hewitt has investigated in detail the French diet for sex selection and has made out diet sheets adapted to provide a nutritionally balanced diet of English foodstuffs which are readily available in the UK. He is currently working on an 'Asian diet' designed to help those who eat predominantly Asian food.

Mr Hewitt carefully follows up his clients to make sure there are no medical complications. He asks you to start by filling in a form detailing your medical history. For £70, you can receive information on his strict diet for either sex of child (*see page 142*). It is tough and, to me, daunting, but there for the taking, if you want to commit yourself. Mr Hewitt says: 'I am still not certain how it works but the results to date suggest that it does work – up to an 80 per cent (or thereabouts) level. It is my personal view [*and I would agree*] that the most likely site of action is at the egg/sperm level – at the time of fertilization in the Fallopian tube.' [*'Preferential fertilization' by X or y sperm is an interesting idea.*]

After having two boys, Keith and Joan Parkinson followed Mr Hewitt's diet for a girl. No salt, no coffee and only bottled water – even in tea. It took three months for Joan to conceive. 'The first few days were really hard because everything tasted so bland,' recalls Joan. 'It was a very healthy diet and, as I was cooking for all of us, my husband, Keith, lost a stone in weight!' Sceptical friends had to eat their words when Joan's amniocentesis proved that the diet had worked, when it predicted a daughter. 'We were tickled pink,' said Joan. 'It was awful but, in retrospect, well worth attempting. You don't get anywhere, if you don't try.'

Although I, personally, find the diet superfluous to the timing method, I grant that eating the appropriate fare cannot harm the sex selection endeavour. The right food can only help the swing to the desired sex, just as the alkaline secretion at female orgasm gives an extra aid to the conception of boys (*see page 58, Chapter 8*). The diet method is not 'proven' any more than is my timing and sperm count theory. Again, one can only go by results.

Janet Fikri, the mother of four sons, combined diet with timing when she tried to swing the balance to a daughter.

I had to try anything [wrote Janet]. And when I saw the diet sheet and read about Hazel's timing theory, I decided to try them both.

It is hard to describe all the things I went through: the food and drinks I had to give up while the rest of the family were carrying on as usual; and especially my husband drinking tea and coffee and me only smelling it! But all this didn't matter because, all the time in my mind, I knew I was going to have my daughter in the end. I also charted my temperature to find my ovulation and was very careful to keep intercourse well before it.

My unbelieving husband changed his mind when our daughter, Yasmin, was born in December 1983 – at long last a sister for our precious boys, Ian, Billy, Eden and Zak. Thanks to you, Hazel Phillips, and to the Mother & Baby *magazine where I read the diet. In the near future, I am willing to try this again for another daughter because everything I have done was worth it.*

Janet Fikri

Janet stuck pretty strictly to the diet though she did not cut out white bread completely as the diet recommended. Many women have followed the diet in a half-hearted sort of way, combining it with the right timing. Both Mandy Aylott and Rosetta Antrobus cut out salt for a month or two before conceiving their daughters. Veronica Pincher, 'wasn't very keen to stick to the special diet but preferred to try the timing method. And I'm thrilled to tell you it worked! We now have a delightful little daughter. Grateful thanks.'

Of course, this sort of behaviour does not prove anything about the diet method because these mothers were also carefully following the right timing. Maybe diet helped; maybe it was irrelevant?

With three sons, Caroline Street was a bit more whole-hearted, though not altogether.

I changed my diet radically. I used to drink gallons of strong tea every day, which I cut out. And I ate all the foods mentioned in your book. Thankfully, I conceived in the second month of trying, so I could go back to normal eating. We made love on Day 9 and then my husband had to go away on busines for a few days. When he came back, we used condoms for the rest of the month. Day 9 was obviously close enough because we got a brilliant result! Rebecca has much improved our family. Having had two boys nineteen months apart, the family was very fraught and argumentative. Having a little girl has made us all change our attitude somewhat. A definite improvement, thanks to your methods. Thanks again,

Caroline

But which method brought her Rebecca?

With four boys in her family, Judith Bradley tried the following.

I pin-pointed ovulation by plotting a temperature chart for six months and by keeping a check on the mucus situation. Intercourse took place approximately sixty hours before ovulation occurred. I also used the diet theory for six months and stuck to it as rigidly as possible, using the information in your book.

Yes!! I produced a daughter for my husband and a granddaughter for my mother-in-law and a sister for my sons! Granny is overjoyed to have a 'pink frilly' grandchild to spoil at last. Christy has really completed and rounded off my brood. She was well worth six months of Perrier water, rice pudding, salt-free bread and raspberry pavlova.

Thank you for my Christy!

Judith.

Again, Diet or Timing? Or both?

As we saw in Chapter 5, when Jonathan came to join his brother James, Elaine Clarke unhappily decided that she would probably never have a girl.

Then I found your book in a shop and 'persuaded' my husband that it was worth a try. I desperately wanted a daughter. I immediately noticed that my diet was totally a boy diet: salt with everything (very unhealthy, I know!!). And constant tea, coffee and fizzy drinks. I never had milk in any form, not even yoghurts or milk in drinks. The afternoon after buying Girl or Boy? I changed my diet immediately — and hated every minute of the next five months! But I really did stick to it because there was a very good reason, I hoped.

The milkman wondered what had hit him! I made myself drink milk all the time. The supermarket must have run out of Perrier and there must have been a bread and salt mountain somewhere, from me not eating any.

I found it very difficult to buy products without salt in, find substitutes for bread and salty cheese etc., and I spent a fortune in health food shops. Most of my friends thought I was mad and were not convinced that the diet could make any difference. But I was willing to try anything.

I mention the diet first as I could start that immediately but, from the morning after buying your book, I started charting my temperature as I, too, was convinced about the timing theory. After three months, it was definite. I ovulated on Day 18 of a 36 day cycle. My temperature went up on Day 19. (I had always had a 30 day cycle but never even knew when I ovulated; the boys had just happened!) I used a digital thermometer which was very accurate, and I always took my temperature before I got out of bed in the morning; it soon became a habit.

We used condoms for the first three months and then, on month four, we decided that the days to try (to play it safe) were Days 13 and 15. We would use condoms after that.

Nothing happened for the first four months. In the fifth month, we had a surprise. We only made love on Day 13 and missed Day 15. Disappointed, I assumed nothing would happen that month either. But, amazingly, my period didn't show up and I found I was pregnant! Could it be a girl? I couldn't believe it until Melissa was born. Even after three months, I don't think it has really sunk in yet. It was all due to your ideas and your theory and I want to say a big Thank you as I may never have known about this and may have been a hockey widow to three or more boys by now!

I hope I haven't bored you by rambling on.

Yours with extreme gratitude,

Elaine

P.S. My midwife has now got your book from me as she always has people asking her about girl or boy selection.

P.P.S. I have now gone back to my old diet. Very unhealthy? But a lot happier!!

You may have noticed that all the diet letters are from mothers of boys, who want a girl. Because it is so much more difficult to get the timing for a girl right, I understand the woman's wish to weight everything she can on the girl's side. I think our normal diet with a great deal of salt leans heavily towards the male diet and many women, like Elaine, have to steel themselves to strictly adhere to the girl diet. The difficulty seems to lie mostly in the demand to give up beverages: coffee and tea are rich in potassium; fizzy drinks interfere with the absorption of calcium from the gut. Surprisingly perhaps, large quantities of salt are found in white flour, white bread, breakfast cereals, chocolate and other convenience foods; no doubt because salt is a cheap, tasty filler-in.

I do not find it surprising that housewives like convenience foods whenever possible. It is so marvellous to buy something in the shop complete with directions for quick cooking, put it in the oven while you take your coat off, and it's *ready*! Chocolate and cheese are even better. They just sit there, winking at you and all you have to do is pick them up and eat them. Delicious! (But not for migraine sufferers!)

Furthermore it is not that astonishing that females enjoy tasty dishes. After all, the nursery rhyme tells us that little girls are 'made of sugar and spice and all things nice'. Many women have tried the salt-free diet, found it impossibly bland and given it up in disgust.

Lauretta Withey told me:

I stopped taking salt and coffee and tried a more nutty diet but got fed up with this. So I was eating equally a girl and boy diet when Suzanne was conceived after intercourse four days before ovulation. I still have to keep pinching myself that it is true. My husband passed some important exams last April, but I feel that Suzanne is a much more important achievement. The boys adore her and she is such a placid baby — much different from the boys. She sleeps all night and six hours in the day and, when she is awake, she is a delight.

We are just one big happy family.

Lauretta

Finally, Pat Frith makes no bones about timing versus diet:

Dear Hazel

I don't know whether you remember me writing to you last February. I had two boys and was pregnant again, worried in case I had gone too close to ovulation in trying for a daughter. I conceived the boys 15/16th day and with Nicola, it was Day 11, just one time, one night. The letter you wrote back to me, reassuring me that it would be a girl because we were ahead of ovulation and because of our ages, was right. We had a beautiful daughter on 14 August

1989, and it's all thanks to you, no question about it. It was your method (timing), and I honestly can't thank you enough.

I don't know whether you saw the headlines on TV in September 1989, about the couple in Liverpool who, after trying for twelve years for a family, had a baby by In Vitro Fertilisation (IVF), the first in Britain. Well, the doctor who did it was Dr Jon Hewitt, the same doctor my husband and I were under for sex selection through diet; no salt for a girl.

He wrote to me last week (October 1989), to find out what I had had and what diet we were on. It may have helped, cutting the salt out, but we think it was the timing. Anyway, Hazel, write back and let me know, please.

Thanks again. God bless you,

Pat and Stan Frith

So, Diet or Timing? Or both? Take your pick and help yourself.

CHAPTER 14

GETTING IT WRONG – IN MISS-CONCEPTION

I will start this chapter on a personal note of sorrow and regret. Then I will consider some early examples of some disappointed mothers who were unsuccessful in getting the child of their choice. I turn to philosophy for guidance on what, if anything, can be done. Then, we will look at other, unhappy cases and see how a remedy may help other mothers in distress.

I extend my deep sympathy to all couples for whom my method of sex selection has not worked. You have a wretched feeling of exasperated impotence when your body produces what you did not choose, don't you? I, too, get that cold feeling in my stomach again when a sad letter arrives with not the best news. You get such ambivalent feelings at the moment of birth that you don't know whether to laugh or cry. I apologize for leading you full of hope up the garden path, as it were, only to double your disappointment in the end. I don't pretend to have all the answers; my method just seems to swing the balance in the desired direction for most people who get the rules exactly right.

My only comfort is that you are not any worse off than if you had not tried my theory. The outcome would probably have been the same. Though I admit that you probably had to fall from a higher pinnacle of hope after my intervention. Your cries of 'What can I do?' ring in my ears, and I feel sad and frustrated too. I have no remedy yet for all the exceptions that prove the rule. But here are a few thoughts on the problem.

Some disappointments are due to mistaken timing and can easily be explained. This tragic letter came from Queensland, Australia. Tragic because the outcome was an unnecessary mistake.

I have two boys [wrote Jessica]. *One is eight and the other five and I can't have any more after this one as I have a small pelvis and cannot have them normally. I sent to a doctor in England for recipes on choosing the sex of babies, and he sent back your recipe. The next month, I tried it.*

I have a 28 day cycle and my period lasts for five days. We had sex on the 6th, 8th and 11th day after my period.

Well, I had a third boy in which I was very disappointed. The specialists and doctors and nurses told me I cried all the way back from the theatre which I don't remember. I really believed all the way, and thought I was carrying a girl because I carried the boys so different: low instead of high, and I was sick on and off. I checked and checked and carried out every little detail. And I was wrong. Could I have made a mistake somewhere? And is there any way that I could find out what it is? I am so upset, as I really wanted a girl.

What's hurting me so much is that I had my tubes tied, as the doctors advised. I've had nightmares ever since. I was very depressed while in hospital and I lost all my milk through crying and not being able to think. Now that I'm home and have had time to think, I love my little boy so much. He's a lovely little boy and I call him David Roger.

Thank you for your letter and kind words. What I look forward to now, is that they grow up to be good lads and able to get a career.

Thanking you,
Jessica

Poor brave Jessica! Can you spot her mistake? She counted wrongly like Helen (*see page 105, Chapter 11*). They both started counting the days from the *end* of their period instead of from the beginning. Day 1 is the first day of bleeding and you must count from there. That was Jessica's only mistake and it cost her dear. If you add on five days to Days 6, 8 and 11, intercourse took place on Days 11, 13 and 16; all round ovulation and just right for a boy.

Pin-pointing ovulation proved to be my stumbling block [wrote Jackie from Kent. She felt she had been cheated of her girl by her fickle, irregular cycle varying between 31–34 days.]

Two years after our first son was born, we decided to try for another baby, hopefully a girl. Being an avid Mother & Baby reader, I spotted your article in that and thought I had nothing to lose by giving it a go. My husband, who I thought would dismiss the idea, agreed with the science of your theory and was happy to support me.

My temperature usually rose sharply on Day 19 and so I reckoned my ovulation to be on Day 19. [No, ovulation occurs just before the high temperature is reached; Day 18 would be more likely, or even Day 17.] *For six months, we played it safe and stopped unprotected intercourse on Day 12. Nothing happened.* [A bit too long before ovulation?] *Then we got fed up* [I am not surprised!] *and decided to continue up to Day 17* [too near] *assuming ovulation to be on Day 19* [mistaken]. *I fell pregnant straight away but unfortunately miscarried* [with a girl? see page 105, Chapter 11]. *After a couple of months, we tried the magic Day 17 again. I again fell pregnant immediately and felt sure I had conceived a daughter.*

I won't lie and tell you that I wasn't disappointed on being told I had produced another son, but that feeling was only momentary and my husband and I soon adored him. However, I still would like another baby; I have always wanted three children. So I have started to chart my cycle again in an effort to pin-point ovulation more accurately. I feel that in order to do this, I will have to invest in one of the more sophisticated devices mentioned in your book, like Ovin. Although, as you state, this is quite costly at £50. However, I feel that this is a small price to pay. Convincing my husband of this will be the problem! [Ovin is no longer available, I'm afraid. Dr Ash, its inventor, died of old age last year. Use modern Ovulation Kits instead.]

Regarding other methods of sex choice, I have to say that I do not have any faith in the diet theory. I eat a vast amount of dairy products, wholemeal bread and, in fact, all the foods listed as forbidden for boys. And I never take salt on my meals or use it in my cooking. [I agree with you; I'm convinced that timing and sperm count are more relevant than diet.]

I passed on your tips to four of my friends who were quite interested and, although they didn't follow the rules rigidly, with temperature charts etc., they made mental notes regarding intercourse timing. I am happy to report that each one of them was successful! It was a constant source of amusement to them that I, who was hardly away from my thermometer and charts, had failed. I enclose a copy of the chart which brought my son.

Thanks again, Hazel, for sharing your hunch with me. Maybe, in a couple of years' time, I will be able to announce the birth of a daughter.

Jackie Brook

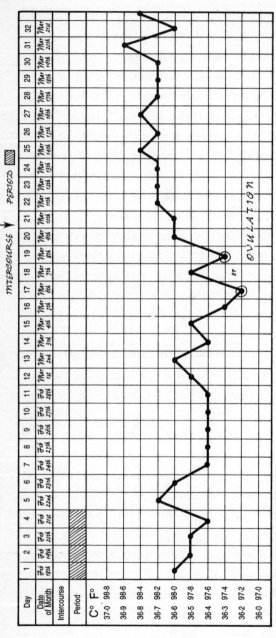

INTERCOURSE ↓   PERIOD ▨

Day	1	2	3	4	5	6	7	8	9	10	11	12	13	14	15	16	17	18	19	20	21	22	23	24	25	26	27	28	29	30	31	32
Date of Month	Feb 18th	Feb 19th	Feb 20th	Feb 21st	Feb 22nd	Feb 23rd	Feb 24th	Feb 25th	Feb 26th	Feb 27th	Feb 28th	Mar 1st	Mar 2nd	Mar 3rd	Mar 4th	Mar 5th	Mar 6th	Mar 7th	Mar 8th	Mar 9th	Mar 10th	Mar 11th	Mar 12th	Mar 13th	Mar 14th	Mar 15th	Mar 16th	Mar 17th	Mar 18th	Mar 19th	Mar 20th	Mar 21st

OVULATION

Fig. 20: Jackie Brook's Chart

Your personal conception charts

1 Insert the date (day and month) at the top of each column in the space provided.

2 Each morning, as soon as you wake up and before you get out of bed, place a thermometer (an ordinary clinical one from any chemist) under you tongue and leave it there for at least two minutes. Do this every morning, including during your period, before you have anything to eat or drink or smoke a cigarette.

3 Record your temperature reading accurately on the chart by making a dot at the appropriate point (see sample chart). If you miss a day, leave a space, and don't join up the dots on either side. Mark the days when you have sexual intercourse with a down-pointing arrow in the space provided.

Use an asterisk to mark any days when you have taken any drugs, including such things as aspirin.

4 The first day of your period is taken to be the first day of your cycle. Indicate each day of menstrual loss by blocking in the square for that day (see sample chart).

5 Any obvious reasons for a change in temperature, such as a cold, insomnia, an infection and so on, should be noted on the graph above the reading for that day.

6 If you feel a twinge of pain in your lower abdomen on ovulation day, mark this on the graph.

7 Start your next cycle on a new chart.

I wrote this letter back to big-hearted Jackie:

Dear Jackie

First of all, congratulations on the birth of your second son! You are in right Royal tradition (1987), aren't you? I am so glad he arrived safe and sound.

Yet I'm very sorry he didn't turn out to be the girl you were hoping for. You must have felt very fed up and cheated after all your careful planning. But I think you have proved my method only too well! I have marked on your beautiful chart [opposite] where I think you ovulated – Day 17 or Day 19! Did you not experience any slippery vaginal mucus on one of those days when the temperature dropped before the sharp rise on Day 18 or Day 20? In tricky cycles like yours you have to go by the mucus. Even if ovulation did not occur until Day 19, intercourse on Day 17 was too close for your fertile husband with a high sperm count.

Maybe your psychological excitement at the prospect of conceiving a girl caused you to ovulate early that month? (It was probably your friends' casual attitude which helped them to succeed where you failed.)

Actually, I think part of your trouble may lie with your husband. I have been working recently on an addition to my theory, connected with sperm count. I have a suspicion that this may be significant in sex determination. I enclose a copy of my research so far.

You seem to have a pretty fertile husband with two sons; he may need to lower his sperm count temporarily to beget a daughter. You must wear him out with heat and sex in the first part of the month! If he can get it low enough, you are bound to have a girl (See Chapter 9).

As I said, Ovin is now unavailable, but there are Ovulation Kits on the market (see page 78, Chapter 9) which give warning of its imminent arrival. When the colour appears, start looking for the slippery mucus that denotes ovulation. Rely on observation of this personal change. And remember that Day 17 is much too dangerous for you to creep up to. I think Day 15 would be a safer stopping place.

When you want to conceive again, send me copies of three or four consecutive temperature charts and I will advise you precisely as to when to make love for your daughter.

Meanwhile, enjoy your bouncing boys. And please congratulate your friends. They can congratulate you next time! And keep up your good humour in face of adversity. That is the best recipe for success!

Best wishes to you all,

Hazel

This sort of letter is a sad but straightforward mistake in timing. Both Jessica and Jackie unfortunately followed the rule for a boy, and inevitably got one.

Other mothers have been disappointed by erratic ovulation too. Sometimes ovulation occurs unexpectedly early so that intercourse takes place on the day of ovulation instead of ahead. Ovulation is not immovably fixed and can easily be thrown out of gear. Violent female orgasm has been known to trigger ovulation as has the psychological pressure on a woman too keyed up to conceive her daughter or son. So, if you ever get the ovulatory mucus at unexpected times, *don't* have unprotected sex unless you want a boy! You need to be exact about the day, as Linda found to her cost (*see page 53, Chapter 7*).

Quite soon after results began to come through my letter box fifteen years ago, a letter of a very different kind arrived to shake me considerably:

Dear Mrs Phillips

I have read your ideas in Mother & Baby *magazine. I have tried out this theory and was unsuccessful. After taking my temperature for nine months, I was certain of my actual ovulation day. I am sure I conceived on the actual ovulation day. Nine months later I gave birth to my third daughter.*

Since having my third child, I have been very depressed. But I and my husband don't dare try again for a boy in case it's another daughter. My children are nine years, seven years and ten months.

Please let me know if you can give me any advice.

Yours sincerely,

Sunita Kaur

I was also depressed – and shocked. This was the first time my theory had been so adamantly refuted. My naive confidence was shaken. Was it all a terrible mistake? Was I wrong to lead people on in expectation only to dash their hopes at the end? The method had worked for me and for my local friends and relations, but did this justify me in putting it forward as a reliable theory? I eventually wrote an apologetic and consoling letter to Sunita Kaur and retreated into the philosophy course I was reading with the Open University. At first this did not help at all.

The erudite philosopher, Sir Karl Popper, was very strict about theories. If you have a theory about something which is then falsified (proven not true), you must discard that theory in favour of a better rival one. There is no room for theories which have been falsified; you cannot draw any more knowledge from them.

If the conclusions have been falsified, then their falsification also falsifies the theory from which they were logically deduced. (Popper, p.33)

What did this say to me as I huddled cringing from a letter which seemed to falsify my theory of sex determination? What should I do? Was my theory wrong? Must I discard it? Surely, there must be some way to counter my and Sunita's failure? Could we not learn from our mistakes?

In despair, I turned to another philosopher, Thomas Kuhn, who was a contemporary of Popper's but who took a very different approach to theorizing. Instead of throwing out a theory which had been refuted, Kuhn staunchly defended his paradigm while he accumulated more knowledge that could improve the theory. Eventually perhaps, the modified theory would be able to withstand all attacks on its veracity?

Scientific enquiry should replace the familiar falsification procedures which end in the rejection of a theory. Rather, new research may accumulate further knowledge to confirm it. (Kuhn, p.8)

Popper and Kuhn had a great debate over their differing attitudes. Popper tested hypotheses by proving them wrong (falsification). Kuhn tried to prove them right through more knowledge (confirmation).

To me, Kuhn's approach appealed. With relief, I followed his advice by delving further into research in another aspect of sex determination: sperm count. I soon found the reason for Sunita's problem. I suggested her husband should get a sperm count taken. This he did, and it was found to be low, thus confirming the prospect of female offspring. Surely this physiological fact would help to take the sting out of Sunita's failure?

With this in mind, I wrote finally to Sunita.

Dear Sunita

Congratulations on the birth of your daughter! I am so glad she turned up safely to join her sisters. They must be a trio of dark-eyed beauties!

But I am very sorry she did not turn out to be the son you worked so carefully for. It must have been a bitter blow when all your efforts came to nought. I apologise for giving you false hope, which must have increased your disappointment.

I'm sorry that I had not done my recent research into sperm count when Girl or Boy? was published. I belatedly enclose this now. And it is a pity I did not know then about your husband's sperm count. Natural misfortunes like that quickly dispose of any plans we might make. But at least you know now that the situation is nobody's fault. You both did all you could to swing the balance to the other sex. But we are helpless against the fixed laws of genetic heredity. It is hard that that has deprived you of the son you wanted so much. I send you my deepest sympathy.

Now, you can settle down with your very attractive family, all of whom are healthy and vigorous. That in itself is something to be proud of. At least you know now why you have your lovely daughters – and that you are not accountable.

Commiserations to your husband too. Don't let him fret about his genetic make-up. That is as futile as wishing for black eyes instead of brown! His potency has been proved beyond doubt by his large family.

Love them and enjoy them as they grow up. No doubt, they will gladden your old age, one day!

Best wishes to you all,

Hazel

I was encouraged to hear from an intelligent couple who followed Kuhn's philosophy instinctively. Naren and Madha had made the common mistake with First Response Ovulation Kit in taking the colour change to *be* ovulation. Like Yasmin (*see page 5, Chapter 1*) they made love too soon and got a 'superb' daughter, Roshni, instead of the first-born son they were hoping for. Far from giving up in disgust and throwing out the theory of sex selection which had not delivered straight away what they wanted, they determined to study it even more carefully and discover where their mistake lay. Perhaps with greater confidence, they would get it right next time?

They revised again every aspect of the theory. They changed their ovulation kit to the simpler one of Clearplan and read the instructions *carefully*. They kept accurate temperature charts for another ten months. They further studied the vaginal mucus. Naren adjusted his sperm count with coolness and abstention after consulting me about the details. They ran a trial month without attempting conception. Then on the day after ovulation when the slippery mucus was copious, they made love for their son.

Naren wrote me this letter:

Dear friend Hazel,

How are you? Guess what? We did a pregnancy test a day after the missed period and it showed positive. We waited a fortnight before going to the doctor for confirmation. Now we can safely say we expect the new arrival on 14 December 1990.

Roshni is ecstatic. She even accidentally told my sister-in-law that we were going to have a baby before the doctor's confirmation and before we had officially told our family!

Hazel, why is there always this waiting? First we were waiting for the mucus pattern; then for the day of ovulation; then waiting for the period to be hopefully repressed; then the pregnancy confirmation. Then the long wait to see the new arrival.

Hazel, it doesn't matter whether it's a boy or girl, but what a wonderful surprise it would be, if it turned out to be a boy. We would like to take this opportunity of thanking you for all your help and support. We want you to keep in touch and let us know any developments. We are still thinking of writing a book with you. What do you think?

Love and kind regards to you from us and Roshni and also our timely arrival,

Naren

Many others of my readers seem to have had similar feelings during the wait of pregnancy! In my experience, much of life is a waiting game. On 8 December 1990 baby boy Methul was born! I had a happy Christmas card from the whole family.

We can never forget you, Hazel. Every time we look at our children, we remember you. (Do you remember our endless correspondence and panic phone calls?) What about a revised book? We could write it together. [Here it is!]

Best wishes for ever and always,
Naren, Madhu, Roshni and Methul

So, Naren and Madhu proved the worth of Kuhn's philosophy of eventual success through further learning and effort!

Other sad letters drove me to redouble my efforts at 'accumulating more knowledge' which might extend the use of my theory to more people. The suffering underlying the following stories makes this chapter hard to write – and to read. Despair makes mothers eloquent and their poignant letters bring a lump to my throat, still. A woman from the North of England wrote me many such letters. Here are two: one of mixed emotions when she was pregnant but scared that she had made a mistake, and another when the worst had happened.

Dear Hazel

Hello. How are you? It's been a long time since I wrote to you. I haven't forgotten you. I've been very busy working and running to and from the school of my daughter, Rani.

Hazel, I'm pregnant! You are the second person to know. My husband was the first. I'm only two months gone yet. We did it [had intercourse] on Day 12, and I just hope this was the right time. I worry so much that we might have done it before ovulation. I don't want to keep going through this over and over again until I have a boy. (Indian families keep at you until you have a boy.)

Hazel, my younger cousin has just had a little boy, thanks to your theory. Everyone kept on that we are older than them and we should try for a boy. (I haven't told anyone yet that I am pregnant.) Rani went to see the baby and she saw my cousin change the nappy. She came back home and said, 'Mum, I think I should have a little baby brother with a tail.'

Hazel, I feel so miserable. I envy my cousin. It's almost as if I am jealous of her having a little boy. She and her husband keep on that they didn't mind, if it was healthy. But I know that my cousin was miserable all through her pregnancy in case she had another girl. And now she looks so happy. All the time, I knew how she was feeling although she would never admit she really wanted a boy. Now I feel the same; I'm so scared. If I have another girl, everyone is going to say I take after my mum. My mum kept having girls.

My husband says it doesn't matter because we can always try again. But I don't really want to have a big family. There are too many unwanted children in the world already. I pray every day; I hope we can have a little boy.

Hazel, I hope you don't mind me keeping writing to you. Please let me know if you get fed up. I feel you are the only person in this world who could really understand how I feel.

Hazel, if I had the choice, I would go to that Clinic in London that separates sperms but my husband does not believe in things like that. He says it is not natural. Even if he has ten girls, he wouldn't go there.

Hazel, my husband has got four brothers and they have all got boys and girls. My husband is the only one who hasn't got a boy. I feel so bad about it. I'm sure my husband feels the same but he would never admit it. He never says he wants a boy and yet he went along when I said I wanted to try your method, Hazel. These nine months are going to be the longest in my life.

Hazel, even if I have a girl, I'll never forget that you were there for me in my bad times when I was feeling really down. I am grateful for your friendship. I know you are busy but I hope you would write to me even if it's only once in 6– 9 months. I have lots of friends but I couldn't open my heart to them.

Love,
Leah Patel

A letter like this makes me very sad. Why must we be so private and superior even to our friends? So that Leah had no one in whom to confide her hopes and fears? Rivalry and one-upmanship in families can be very cruel. Would not friendly discussion and sympathy make everyone a lot happier? It doesn't make the likelihood of choosing the sex of *your* baby any more or less, if you are mindful of someone else along the way! In fact, it would probably increase the celebration at the birth – or the condolence, if that were sadly required.

I immediately wrote back to Leah, saying that of course she was jealous of her cousin. She wouldn't be human if she were not! But be patient for a bit longer and maybe you won't need to feel jealous any more. I pointed out that neither she nor her mother deserved blame for bearing daughters. It takes two to produce a child and people who exclusively blame the woman for the sex, just show their ignorance (*see page 25, Chapter 5*). As we saw there, the unchosen sex of a baby is nobody's *fault*. With Leah's mother, the row of girls *was* probably due to ignorance of any remedy. If Leah had now made a mistake, it would be even more tragic, as she had tried so hard to follow the rules for her son. Her temperature record was good and she had made love at the midmonth drop on Day 12. But had she made love *before* her ovulatory pain? And the slippery mucus?

Seven months later, this letter arrived:

Dear Hazel,

I have given birth to a little girl. It seems your method does not work for me. In a 24–26 day cycle, we abstained from sex until night 12. I ovulate on Day 11 or 12 every month. Don't get me wrong. I love my second little girl the same as I love my first, but I'm heart-broken. I feel as if I've lost my last hope on this earth to have the little boy I've always wanted. It took me six years to go for another child and now I've even lost my last hope.

I hope you don't mind me writing to you. You are the only one I opened my heart to even before I got pregnant. I was looking forward to this baby, hoping and praying it'll be a brother for my daughter.

I went through so much pain and I've had so many stitches I can hardly move. At times like this, I wish I wasn't Indian. God knows how many times I'll have to try before I get a boy. I just can't take the labour pains and the sleepless nights. I cry every day. The worst thing is that all my husband's brothers have boys. Out of all his brothers, he is the only one who doesn't have a son. I feel I let him down, let myself down. For Indian men it's different. If one wife can't give them a son, they get married again and everybody understands. I didn't want a big family and I don't want to keep trying for a boy. The pressure is on me even though it's the man's sperm that decides if it's a boy or a girl.

Maybe there is something wrong with me? Maybe my body only accepts female sperms? I feel so depressed. I wish the ground would open up and swallow me. I never want to go out now.

Sorry about the writing so scruffy. I thought I'd let you know what I've had.

Love,

Leah

How could I answer that? I was torn in two, along with Leah. With my heart bleeding, I wrote:

My dear Leah

What a sad, sad letter! And now you have such discomfort and pain to add to your terrible disappointment. This just adds insult to injury. I am so sorry. You must have been absolutely devastated when another girl appeared – after you had tried so hard to swing the balance to a boy. You must find nature very cruel and unfair.

Nature is cruel in many ways. But she is fair in the game of sex selection. She has definite rules and, if we keep to them precisely, we get the child we want. The trouble is that it is so easy to make a mistake.

I was looking through our previous correspondence and found a letter from you in which you said you were worried that you may have made love before you ovulated that month. Maybe this was so? Did you have intercourse before you experienced your ovulatory pain and the slippery mucus? It is very hard but you have to be absolutely accurate in obeying nature's rules. Just hoping for the best will not do. If you followed the intercourse-before-ovulation rule for a girl, a girl turned up in true consequence.

What can I say to comfort you? Only that the method did work for you although you made a mistake. Being human, we all make mistakes but this sort is very costly. I am so sorry it happened.

But your temperature chart for the month in which you conceived your second daughter was good. From that, it would seem that you did make love right on Day 12, the day of ovulation. Next day, Day 13, your temperature rose sharply to the higher post-ovulatory level. If you made love on the day of ovulation and still got a daughter, it may be that your husband's sperm count was too low on that day to beget a son. I would recommend that he have a sperm count taken. Then, at least, you would know why you conceived a second daughter and if it is worth trying again for a son. I wouldn't want you to go through another birth, if there was no hope of a boy.

If your husband's sperm count is congenitally low, there is no point in trying over and over for a boy. Low sperm count generally produces a girl. But if his sperm count is normal usually and just happened to be low on the day you tried for a boy, he may be able to raise it with appropriate treatment (see page 82, Chapter 10). If he gets a sperm count taken, let me know the result and we will see if there is a chance of changing it.

Your husband could get a sperm count done for £25 by contacting one of these Marie Stopes Clinics:

Marie Stopes Centre	or	Jeff Mitchell
1 Police Street		60 Wimpole Street
Manchester M2 7LQ		London W1M 7DE
Tel: 0161 832 4260		Tel: 0171 487 4644
		Ring on Wednesday morning.
		Dr Mitchell works for the
		London Marie Stopes Centre, W1

I am afraid you (and I) will suffer wretched pangs of regret over the next few months. You will have the anguished yearning of 'If only . . .' every time you see the happy mother of a son – like your cousin. But try not to let that feeling spoil everyone's enjoyment of him and of your new daughter. It will take a lot of courage but you will feel better if you are frank and honest about the new *births in the family. Say to your cousin, 'You lucky thing! We tried so hard to get a boy too, but we made a mistake and here is Rani's sister to prove that we were not as clever as you! But she is a sweet little thing, isn't she? And maybe we will get things right next time. We'll have to, as large families are so expensive and exhausting.'*

And, in your case, Leah, so painful. Spend some time coddling yourself and your new baby. Get to know her and enjoy her first smile! The next weeks will be hard for you both – and for your husband who sounds so level-headed and supportive.

If you want to try again in a few years, write to me before you start and we'll make sure you get everything right. I'll talk you through, step by step, as I am doing for another woman right now. She wants a boy too and I'll tell you how she gets on.

Congratulations on surmounting the difficult birth of your daughter. Now you have two dark-eyed beauties! Love to you all,

Hazel

What about other women who *know* they got all the timing absolutely right and yet conceived another son? In my experience, there have been six such cases every year since 1987. I also have sleepless nights over these boys – as well as their mothers!

My growing investigation into sperm count show how imperative it is to keep intercourse as far away from ovulation as possible when trying for a girl. Especially, if you have a fertile husband with sons already. One such man seems to be the husband of Maribel of South London.

Trying meticulously to conceive a daughter, Maribel and her husband, John, thought they had followed all the rules to the letter. They stopped intercourse two days before ovulation. When she became pregnant, Maribel hoped and believed she was carrying a girl. But, after a painful confinement, out came another boy – to the disbelief of his parents. And no doubt, to the pleasure of his brother, Tom.

In her mid-thirties, Maribel feared that her time for getting a daughter was running out. (But that is one point on which I can reassure her, say I. My mother was forty-five when I was born, her fifth child!)

The incidence of female births rises with the age of the parents as all bodily processes, including the production of sperm, diminish with age.

Both Maribel and her husband rang me to break the happy/sad news of the birth, and they asked frantically what to do. After welcoming their bonny baby into the world, my advice was this:

Try and forget all about baby girls for a while. Don't rush into hasty action. Get to know and enjoy your fine sons while your initial disappointment fades a little. Watch your boys learning to be pals. And enjoy their differences! You have a bonus in your second son, especially from the boys' point of view. Many males are sensitive creatures and often less self-sufficient than females. Although unfortunately, it means a bigger family, lots of boys benefit from the solidarity that a brother can provide. A brother can help him to face some of life's perplexing events, especially in adolescence, with the manly, cool courage so often expected of him, still. Such a stiff upper lip is often not demanded of women; we are allowed to take refuge in tears!

So, John and Maribel, bide your time for a couple of years and get your sons off to a flying start. Then you can try again, keeping intercourse well before ovulation. Make your plan about when to stop and then forget about baby girls. Return to honeymoon days and make love for the pleasure of it, thinking about each other rather than babies. The more relaxed the atmosphere, the better. Then see if the boys' sister will surprise you one day to give you the lovely family of two boys and a girl. Please let me know when she arrives!

Hazel

Two and a half years later, a scan predicted the coming of *twin* sons! What a feat! What a family! What fertility! Congratulations! This time John and Maribel had stopped three days before ovulation, but no sign of a girl. Apparently, even three days was not enough to kill off all fecund John's vigorous androsperm. Initially, the scan's verdict came as a bitter blow to the parents who had tried so longingly to introduce their family to the delights of girls. But it was not to be. With a somewhat heavy heart, I tried to console them.

Dear Maribel

Your phone call this morning stabbed my heart, as did your heartbroken words. I imagine myself in your situation and it's unthinkable! All you wanted was a little girl and you end up with four sons. Fate or nature must seem very cruel. I am so sorry.

But there is no personal vindictiveness involved. The natural system has fixed rules for sex selection and, if we don't conform to them exactly, we don't get the child of our choice. The trouble is that for some of us it is so hard to obey them precisely. Stopping three days before ovulation would be all right for a girl in most cases. But with a fertile couple like you and John, a longer time has to elapse between intercourse and ovulation. Young and fertile, I conceived both my girls after intercourse 5 days before ovulation.

I didn't really want to get pregnant then because my husband had just been posted to Crail in Scotland to do his National Service in the Navy and I was scared of being pregnant the first time so far from home. We had thought we were in the 'safe' period, as Day 5 was straight after a period. I didn't know, in those days, how short a cycle I had (24 days only with ovulation on Day 10). So Day 5, five days before ovulation, was just right for a girl, though I would probably have chosen a boy first! But that is how it goes. However strong, wishful thinking has no power in sex selection. The rule prevails!

It was worse for you because you and John had tried to follow the rules. So ultimately, events turned out to be my fault because I hadn't warned you how long fertile androsperm can survive. I'm very sorry. In your vexation, it is natural to look for a scapegoat, but you must not blame your poor husband, Maribel. Poor chap! He must have felt frustrated too, when he learned about the twins. I should think he is almost as miserable as you, since all his devotion seems unable to give you the daughter you crave. So now you are both in the same boat of disappointment. You need to pull together to get out of this trough.

My own grandmother suffered like you. Married at eighteen, she was the second wife to a Victorian gentleman who had three sons already. My grandmother soon produced three more sons. She hoped and hoped for a daughter. When she fell pregnant again she prayed and prayed for a daughter. (A bit late to change things then!) She ended up, like you, with twin sons! As was customary in those days, one of the twins died but my grandmother turned to face the future and moulded her seven surviving sons into a happy and successful family. And in no time at all, as it seemed twenty years later, she was the matriarch of a vast clan of seven brothers with six brides. The second son never married but looked after their mum to the end of her life.

Although, like her, you will always miss a daughter. But I think you have the guts to make the best of things, as my grandmother did. At the moment you *probably feel bitter and melancholy. But this situation is paradoxical when you set it against the many women who are struggling to have a healthy baby at all! There is always someone worse off than you. This reminds me of Pollyanna's Glad Game which I read about years ago, in my youth. Eleanor Porter's story is typical of the Victorian morals on which I was brought up and some of which stick in my mind to this day.*

Pollyanna was the daughter of a poor missionary in Africa (as I was once). Churches back in the home country used to collect oddments of toys and jumble and send out as parcels to the children of such missionaries. Pollyanna longed for a doll. She waited in hope and expectancy. When the parcel arrived, Pollyanna opened it to find – a pair of crutches. Father comforted his sobbing daughter and said, 'Well anyway, you can be glad you don't need them.'

From then on, Pollyanna always looked for something to be glad about in any disaster that befell her. I recommend the Glad Game to all who face deep disappointment. It helps. And below, Maribel and John seem to be playing it!

But I too was sad and vexed. Was Popper right after all? Hanging on to a falsified theory would bring much frustration and heartache to unfortunate parents who had had the lure of hope dangled before their eyes. Perhaps I was mistaken to go on trying in the face of such setbacks? Then I had a lesson from Maribel herself.

Today, I rang Maribel to see how the family was getting on now that the twins were nine months old. Dinner time was nearing and bedlam reigned in the background! A harassed but cheerful Maribel answered the phone and I could hear the calming tones of father John soothing the vociferous younger members of his large brood.

The twins? [Maribel told me.] Oh yes, they're beautiful! A real handful, of course, and I never stop! But the saving grace is that they are good at night and sleep right through.

During my hectic days, I often imagine how I would feel if they were girls. Right on top of the world! It didn't happen. And now we've got four of them and all I ever wanted was a little girl! Still, and for ever, my soul cries out for a daughter. But, however much we tried, it was not to be because of the mistakes we both made: I didn't persist enough in leaving adequate time between intercourse and ovulation. And John didn't persist enough with the jock-strap.

Hey-ho! But the boys are a great crowd and we are lucky to have them. We would not swap them now. Maybe – if we hit the jackpot . . . we might try again . . .?

This sort of cheerful acceptance always moves me. I come across courage like this repeatedly. It is hard for anyone who has not experienced it, to imagine a woman's feelings of indignant frustration when she cannot get her body to produce what she chooses. And the same goes for the man too. It seems so unreasonable that you cannot make your body do what you want. (It is a bit like having MS!) Saddled with a job for life not quite of their choosing, these admirable parents love and cherish the children of their loins although they are denied the variation of a different sex which would make all their work seem new and different. Nevertheless, many such mothers and fathers of single sex progeny bring up their families to be among the greatest I know. Congratulations to them!

Belinda from Kent wrote with news of her third son after she had tried for a girl by stopping two days before ovulation. 'I was disappointed but I discovered the sex at a 19 week scan and so had time to get used to the idea before he arrived.'

This seems to me a good idea, so that emotional equilibrium can be regained before the birth and the child can receive the welcome it deserves.

You may remember that, at the beginning of this book, I referred to both our daughters as 'mistakes', albeit the best mistakes we ever made. Fortunately, they *seem* (?) to have forgiven me this gaffe. In fact, it soon became quite a joke within the family. These two daughters had turned up because I, in those days, did not know about the significance of the timing of intercourse in sex determination. But these mistakes lay in my lack of planning before conception; *not* in the adorable ducklings who turned into such beautiful and happy swans and who rapidly became a delight to everyone's heart. And you can see what beneficial consequences followed from my 'mistakes'. Without them, this book would never have been written!

Of course, once the baby is born, there must be *no* talk of mistakes, even in jest. I am not sure if my behaviour all those years ago was of the best; children can often read more than you imagine into jocular remarks that can colour their outlook on the world for a long time. The baby must be welcomed as the unique human being it is. And no doubt, a winsome one as well!

The final word goes to sanguine Joanne Millar as she hugged her third son. *Jake is a treasure and we love him and his brothers to bits. We wouldn't swap them, but something's still missing in our lives. Next year, we are off for a holiday abroad and we'll decide if we'll have a fourth! If so, I'll be in touch!! I would still love a daughter to be a friend later on in life. We shall see!*
Love from

Joanne and Andrew, Jamie, Jonathan and Jake

P.S. December 1995. I have just had a Christmas card and letter from Joanne. Spurred on by the recent success of her friend, Gaynor (see page 106, Chapter 11), she is embarking on her fourth attempt to get a daughter. She will have all the help that I can give and I hope she will be as happy as Gaynor. Her resolve and careful planning deserve success. Good luck to her!

Stop Press! This letter from Angela Geraghty has just arrived. I think it is worth putting in; it speaks for itself.

Hi Hazel

Remember me and my three girls? I had my baby on 27 February. I had a little girl. She is lovely. She weighed 9lb 15½ oz, nearly ten pounds.

I am not disappointed. She is very cute. Well, I timed everything right so it seemed to me I am not to have a son. For some reason known to God above. We now have four children and can't afford any more. So I am now to forget about having a son. Hazel, why do women feel they need to have a son to feel complete? Did you feel complete when you had your son? Did he make a difference? Please be honest. Does having what you want and haven't got make you happy or do we only think it does? I feel at the moment that I want to be happy with what I've got, but people keep taking it away when they see my new cute baby girl. They all say. 'Oh, you have to go again for your son?' I feel like saying, 'No, I don't have to go again.' Do you understand? When I was pregnant I went to a fortune teller. She told me I would have a son. But I feel at the moment maybe I am not missing much in not having a son. I think maybe because of my childhood. I had a hard childhood because of my older brother. He was the only son for years. He was spoilt.

My mother had four girls before she had her second son. So my older brother was the only boy for a very long time. He got everything. If I was talking to my mother and my brother walked in to the room I would be forgotten about. He would break windows and doors if he didn't get his own way and Mummy would not tell Dad who did it and we would be put to bed. This went on for years.

I think sometimes I only wanted a son to prove I would treat him the same as my girls. Does that make sense to you Hazel? I know you will write to me and tell me what you think. I know you are a very positive person, and thank you for all your support last year. I will never forget you.

Yours faithfully
Angela Geraghty

My dear Angela

Congratulations on the birth of your daughter! I am so glad Alicia turned up safe and sound to join her sisters. She must complete a bevy of beauties!

But I'm heartbroken that she was not the son you and your husband were hoping for. After all those letters and all the hard work put in both by you and your husband, it is a shame to have a result like this. You tried so hard for a boy and I had great hopes for you after getting your letter last July 1994. When I read your letter today, I nearly wept with disappointment. So what must it have been like for you two?

The vexing sorrow of frustration, I suppose. The same result after all your efforts to swing the balance towards a boy. You must be fed up with me and my theories. I apologize if I made it worse by making you fall from a higher pinnacle of hope.

Tears sprang to my eyes again when I read of your brave acceptance of the situation and the reasons for your wanting a boy. What a sad history of your childhood! That would be enough to give anyone a grudge against men for life! But you don't seem to have any such grudge. Your loving husband must have been instrumental in overcoming it.

Life will be very hard for you both over the next few weeks, when tactless people say the sort of things you report. Here is a hint that may help you to confront them: Don't pretend that you are not disappointed. Say rather, 'Yes, isn't it a wretched quirk of fate, after we had tried so hard to swing the balance? But she is a cute little thing, isn't she? An addition to my bevy of beauties! We just don't seem able to get a boy – must be something to do with my husband's prowess as a drinker in the past.'

This sort of thing will be hard for you to say but, if you can manage it, you will feel better and so will all your friends who are probably embarrassed at your discomfiture. They don't know what to say so it will be better if you can lead the conversation. It will demand a great effort from you. But I am sure it would relieve the tension – and be good for your daughters to hear.

What I say above about your husband's drinking is probably true, I think. He has been so noble recently, staying away from the drink and subjecting himself to all that cold sponging. But I fear that the damage had already been done. The doctors' report in The Lancet says that 'heavy drinking shrivels the testicles and lowers sperm count'. So I fear that your husband's earlier enjoyment of ten pints of beer in one evening out must have lowered his sperm count and been responsible for your daughters. Still, I expect it makes him a happy husband and father, so you can be glad about that!

The only other comfort I can offer you is to point out that an all girl family can be much more interesting than an all boy family, in my opinion. Usually, girls are so diverse in their interests and activities while they are growing up. They can think about things other than football and cars! Of course, it is very sad for your husband that he will have no male ally in the family until his daughters give him some sons-in-law. But that will happen all too soon, I expect!

Meanwhile, stick to your brave acceptance of the healthy family you have produced and enjoy them. Of course you don't have to go on and on for a boy. If you can settle down and be happy with your gorgeous girls, you will be an example to the rest of us who make such a fuss about getting a mixture. Of course, that is what most of us want, but it is not necessary for a fulfilled life. And it is silly and petulant to keep on about something that is impossible. A wise philosopher once said, 'If things are impossible, you stop wishing for them.' Take his advice and enjoy your lovely family. Tell your tactless friends that you know that a son is a lost cause with your macho drinking partner. You know more than they do!

There is a greater courage in accepting your lot gracefully than in constantly kicking bitterly against it. Though I will always rue the fact that you could not put into action your plan of bringing up a son to be kinder than your brother in his childhood. You will have to postpone your mission *for a generation and teach your daughters to bring up their sons aright. Time passes so quickly that you will be a Granny before you can believe it!*

Older cousins of mine had a charming family of girls. The parents were disappointed at having no son to carry on his father's legal business, but sex determination came too late for them. However, I have always looked up to this family as an example of perfectly brought up, fascinating young women. And now the second one has married a qualified lawyer who can engage his father-in-law in legal talk at any time! Now, all married and all with children, some natural, some adopted, the wider family is still a pleasure to know. I'm sure yours will be the same.

Interestingly, one daughter who sadly could not have children of her own, chose to adopt a family of three girls! And she and her husband are making an excellent job of bringing them up. My cousins' experience proves that all is certainly not lost in a single sex family!

Nevertheless, I shall have some sleepless nights along with you in thinking 'If only . . .' The laws of nature can seem very cruel when we don't discover in time how to bend them to our wishes.

I send you both my deepest commiserations and sympathy, as well as my congratulations!

I'm sure the Geraghty Girls will be a foursome to be remembered. Kerry, Samantha, Amy and Alicia will grow up to be blessings to their devoted and caring parents.

My love to you all,

Hazel

And a final postscript from Angela who displays noble sportmanship in losing the game of sex selection:

The way I look at things now is this. All during my pregnancy, I thought I was going to have a son. But during the last three weeks I couldn't see a boy. I felt it was a girl. I can't explain it, Hazel, and sometimes I find the whole thing funny – all the temperature taking and no drinking, and I still got a girl. She is so special to me because I worked so hard before she came. She is worth all the trouble. There is a very special bond between me and my little girl.

I don't feel depressed any more. Maybe it's because I don't want to try again. I have my family now and I'm content. I tried and it didn't work for me, but at least I tried. And now I have a healthy baby at the end. Some people don't have that sometimes. She is healthy and has come to me to be loved and that is what she will get.

I have put your book in a box for my daughters in case they need it one day. We will never forget you.

Angela

Stop Press – Postscript

Wonders never cease. Angela has just announced the arrival of an unplanned 9 lb son, Jason, fifteen months after his youngest sister. Everyone is in shock! *Congratulations!* Now you know, Angela, what it feels like to have the mixed family you wanted.

My 'Kuhn' style explanation would put it down to Angela's new calm psychological state as exemplified in the letter above. She also took a course of reflexology which further relaxed her. So she followed her natural feelings and made love bang on ovulation day with the normal result of a boy.

Looking at Angela's temperature chart for May 1994 when she conceived Alicia, I can be wise in retrospect. Her temperature did not rise to the highest post-ovulatory level until Day 18, indicating that she ovulated on Day 16 or 17. And she had made love at the mid-month drop on Day 12, four or five days before ovulation. No wonder her fourth daughter turned up! To be sure of a boy, wait for the temperature rise. Or be rash and lucky – like Angela!

CHAPTER 15

THE WORLD POPULATION PROBLEM – CHOOSE AND STOP!

'Done because we are too menny.'

(*Jude the Obscure*, part vi, Chapter 2)

———————

This note, written in pencil and in the boy's hand, lay on the floor below Jude's pendent body. Overwhelmed by the crippling poverty of his constantly growing family, the elder boy had hanged his younger siblings and then himself, in a futile attempt to improve the lot of his fecund parents. 'For the rashness of those parents he had groaned, for their ill-assortment he had quaked, and for the misfortunes of these he had died.' (ibid.)

Thus, in 1895, Thomas Hardy described the hopeless poverty trap of those with a surplus of unchosen children, in days of little or no contraception.

The greatest achievement of this book will be in any contribution it makes to checking what I see as the most menacing problem of our time – the population explosion. Few of us could tolerate the extreme action taken by young Jude, or by the Chinese, to solve their population problem. In China, couples are limited to a one-child policy. This often leads to dire consequences. Any further offspring are either aborted, or killed at birth by drowning or lethal injection. Older babies, mostly the less-preferred girls, are abandoned to 'dying rooms' in state orphanages where they die alone from hunger and neglect in conditions which are, as described by a BBC reporter, 'so appalling as to be an affront to humanity.'

But, consider China's predicament. The relentless additions to her vast population portend famine, starvation and death for *everybody* when the population becomes too great for the available land to sustain. Her statesmen are desperate to reduce the population. Chairman Deng Xiaoping is reported to have told his subordinates, 'I don't care how you do it but *do it.*'

This paragraph echoes the premonitions given many years ago by Thomas Malthus, a controversial social philosopher of the eighteenth century. Malthus wrote a book, *Essay on the Principle of Population as it affects the Future Improvement of Society* (1798). In this book, he developed the thesis that human populations, like animal populations, tend to increase in numbers up to the limit of the environment to support them. War, famine and plague ultimately intervene to regulate further growth.

We may weep over the tragedies of Hardy's saga and the Chinese dilemma. Now let us look at the hard facts of the world's situation.

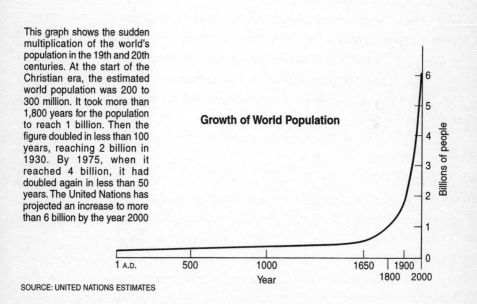

This graph shows the sudden multiplication of the world's population in the 19th and 20th centuries. At the start of the Christian era, the estimated world population was 200 to 300 million. It took more than 1,800 years for the population to reach 1 billion. Then the figure doubled in less than 100 years, reaching 2 billion in 1930. By 1975, when it reached 4 billion, it had doubled again in less than 50 years. The United Nations has projected an increase to more than 6 billion by the year 2000

Growth of World Population

Billions of people

SOURCE: UNITED NATIONS ESTIMATES

Fig. 21: Growth of World Population from AD 1 – AD 2000.

On the previous page is another chart, about girls *and* boys. It traces the population growth of the world from AD 1 to AD 2000. For nineteen centuries, the graph had risen only slowly as men struggled to control the disasters that kept the population down through early death from disease and war. But at the beginning of the twentieth century, the line switched suddenly to the vertical. Why?

War rages still, but a large number of potentially fatal diseases have been conquered in many countries. The sad fact is that the more successful we are in this endeavour, the nearer draws the danger of population saturation. What a pity we did not get the order right and control birth rates before reducing death rates.

Today, medical and technological interventions do two things relevant to this discussion. At the beginning of life they save and succour previously irrecoverable babies born sick or prematurely. In our last years, they extend our lives and push death ever further away as we live longer and longer. As ever, 'a population grows in size if the number of births exceeds the number of deaths. The low death rates that have been achieved are generating rapid population increases.' (James Giesel, Population Growth. p.403 *Encyclopaedia Americana* 1985)

> In his book, *Preparing for the Twenty-first Century*, Paul Kennedy writes:
> *Already, the sheer concentrations of people — 140,000 per square mile in Lagos, Nigeria, and 130,000 in Jakarta, Indonesia — make it inconceivable that their inhabitants will enjoy the benefits offered by affluent cities like New York with a mere 11,400 per square mile. Such imbalances influence how the various races of the globe view one another; they affect international and domestic politics, the social fabric, and the policies of food, energy and migration. Consider the burdens that will be placed on such cities for already inadequate housing, food distribution, sanitation, transport and communications, if their populations double or treble in size. The real challenge will come in the next twenty to forty years, when urbanization in the developing world will exacerbate all these problems associated with high population density, producing miserable living conditions for the vast majority of human beings presently in their infancy or soon to be born.*

Furthermore, not only does the demographic explosion hurt the population's masses. It also does overwhelming damage to resources and the environment, as human beings destroy forests, burn fossil fuels, drain wetlands, pollute rivers and oceans, and ransack the earth for ores, oil and other materials. It is important to gauge the number of people engaged in these activities. In 1975, it was 4 billion; the projected figure for 2025 is 8 or 9 billion. The overall consensus is that, 'The projected growth in the world's population cannot be sustained *with our current patterns and levels of consumption.*' (p.32, Kennedy)

As the environmentalists point out, many of those who pillage the earth's resources are found in the so-called 'civilized' cities of the affluent world. For example, the consumption of oil in the United States – with only 4 per cent of the world's population – equals one quarter of the total world annual production. In 1989, the United States consumed 6.3 billion barrels of oil, hundreds of times more than most third world countries which make do on very little. The average American baby represents 35 times more environmental damage than that of the Indian child because its level of consumption throughout its life will be so much greater.

The earth is therefore under a two-pronged attack from human beings: on the one side are the excessive demands and wasteful lifestyle of wealthy populations in the developed world; on the other appear the ever increasing billions of hungry mouths born in the developing world who, very naturally, aspire to the standard of living enjoyed by the affluent.

The optimists claim that man's inventiveness and technology has an infinite capacity for discovering new resources and keeping ahead of disasters predicted by the modern day Malthus.

Time will tell which viewpoint is correct as the world's population hurtles towards Malthus' dire prediction of 7, 8 or even over 10 billion. If the optimists are right, the world's wealth will be unevenly distributed among the comparatively few prosperous people, with all the insecurity that such a situation engenders. If they are wrong, the ship of human life could founder and sink in a sea of misery.

Unless we seek for an alternative.

At the end of the nineteenth century, just as Hardy was writing, the population graph took off in an exponential curve which rises almost vertically and clearly shows the *doubling* of the world population at regular intervals (*see page 167 of this chapter*). In some parts of Britain, it may be hard to comprehend what that means. But think on this:

The present (1994) population of India is 911.6 million.
By the end of the week, it will have grown by another 3.330846 million.
And every week.
Against that, set the weekly number of deaths =   0.175307 million.
Net increase every week =   3.155539 million.

The present (1994) population of China is 1192 million.
By the end of the week, it will have grown by another 2.521538 million.
And every week.
Against that, set the weekly number of deaths =   0.160461 million.
Net increase every week. =   2.361077 million.

Multiply each of these totals by 52 and the annual increase is more than twice the population of Britain. *Every* year. How can any nation assimilate that?

Some parts of the world are clearly overloaded and in danger of drowning in people. I find this threat to be the most intimidating peril ahead of us. In this global boat, we are all netted together. If one part sinks, the rest must go with it. There will be no winners in the potential scenario of food and land starvation. The panic grabbing of room and space can be seen already in Bosnia and Rwanda, with all the consequent cruelty and suffering.

You think I am exaggerating the threat posed by the growing world population? Listen to the tale of the water lily:

A farmer had a big pond for fish and ducks. On the pond was a tiny lily. It was doubling in size every day. 'Look!' said the people to the farmer. 'You had better cut this back. One day it will be so big that it will kill all your fish and ducks.'

'All right, all right,' said the farmer. 'But there's no hurry. It is only growing very slowly.' The lily carried on doubling in size every day. 'Look,' said the farmer. 'It still only covers half the pond. No need to cut back yet.'

The next day, the farmer had a big surprise.

I feel that the lily of human fecundity is approaching the half-way mark. We have only just begun to cut back. In the past, poor contraceptive methods took the question out of our control. But now we have the choice. I would urge all women to choose their children; then stop! While there is still hope.

Look now at the statistics for Britain and Europe as a whole:

The present (1994) population of Britain is 58.4 million.

By the end of the week, it will have increased by	0.002246 million.
And every *week.*	
Against that, set the weekly number of deaths =	0.012353 million.
Net de-crease every week =	- 0.010107 million.

The present (1994) population of Europe is 728 million.	
By the end of the week, it will have increased by	0.140000 million.
And every week.	
Against that, set the weekly number of deaths =	0.154000 million.
Net de-crease every week =	- 0.014000 million.

How has this reversal of fortunes come about?

In the late 1940s, there was throughout the world a post-war baby boom, as young couples crawled out from the suffocation of war and tried to return to a normal life of love and procreation. The birth-rate soared. It was not long before all observers agreed that the world was facing a population crisis.

Demographers began to give pessimistic forecasts of disasters along the lines predicted by Thomas Malthus. The inevitable sequel after prodigal increase in population was war, famine and plague. 'But,' Malthus had added, 'the moral restraint of abstention and delayed marriage could also regulate further growth.'

This is precisely what happened in the United States and Europe thirty years ago. And the results are now showing. Young people increasingly show a preference for a later age of marriage. This is reflected in my own family. My husband and I were married aged twenty-three and twenty-one respectively. But none of our children was married before the age of thirty

To digress slightly. In some ways, this practice of later marriage is to be regretted, I think. Physiologically speaking, the twenties is the easiest decade for giving birth because the woman is normally then at her optimum, both physically and emotionally, for child-bearing. But as always, economic factors override all competitors, and money is still what makes the world go round. Understandably, young couples prefer to establish themselves economically before plunging into parenthood. But it is known that fertility declines and pregnancy dangers increase as age rises towards thirty and beyond. It seems a pity if economic considerations cause us to pass over this critical point in our reproductive lives.

To return to Malthus' predictions of the consequences of overpopulation. These did not materialize in North America and Europe because of the shift to a later age for marriage and because of the introduction and adoption of fertility control through contraception. The *Encyclopaedia Americana* describes events like this:

> On the one hand, the aroused national leadership of politicians, clerics, universities, medical schools and economic leaders endorsed the importance of slower population growth and urged action to accomplish it. And on the other hand, the mass of people showed overwhelmingly their willingness for such change as they quickly grasped the significance of over-population for themselves and their families. The public eagerly consumed any information about the subject of birth control that was made available to them.

In countries where contraception has been accepted and even embraced with relief, the relentless tide of babies and more babies has been stemmed. We have been given a little breathing space. I hope this book will help to enlarge that gap.

There is abundant evidence that the replacement two-child family is rapidly becoming the cultural norm of the new generations. Especially when the parents are lucky or clever enough to get both sexes in their first two children. When the second child is the same sex as the first, this often means, as it did in my own case, a larger family as the mothers and fathers try again to experience the full potential of parenthood by producing children of both sexes. As you have read, my own grandmother brought up seven sons, while longing for a daughter. If one of those boys had been a chosen girl, her family might have been much smaller.

We have seen how deeply felt is the desire to choose the sex of one's children. No one should be ashamed of such a desire – it is the most natural wish in the world. But we should try to ring the changes with a smaller number of offspring. Safe, harmless and free, the natural method of sex selection is to be recommended.

A few years ago, I took part in a car rally to promote the charity, Population Concern. I quoted Hardy for a slogan on the sides of my car, WE ARE TOO MANY and I used my daughters' doll on the roof to push home the message: OVERPOPULATION IS EVERYBODY'S BABY

Earlier in this book, you will have read that I have an illness for which science has not yet found an answer – Multiple Sclerosis. My own doctor is one of the best and he says frankly to me, 'You know there is nothing I can do for you. No cure. The only thing is management.' And this is what he helps me with, as do all the clever gadgets for the disabled.

How to choose the sex of your baby is also a problem which has not yet been scientifically solved. But, as demonstrated on these pages, choice can be managed if you learn and follow the rules of natural sex selection in a calm and balanced manner, preferably laced with a good dose of humour!

If you can approach it like this, there can be no harm in trying a little 'management' to conceive the child of your choice which would be – in the words of so many of the families who tried and succeeded – the icing on the cake.

RESULTS FOR RESEARCH

If you try this natural method of sex selection, please write to me and let me know the outcome. I love to get letters from you with news of your new baby. You sound so thrilled – it rubs off on me. It is like having another baby – without all the hassle!

I would like to hear of any disappointments too, although they make me sad. Please tell me exactly what you did or didn't do. Every bit of information goes into my research file and, who knows, perhaps I will be able to help you get it right next time?

At least, I can send a letter of consolation and sympathize with your necessarily ambivalent feelings.

Please enclose a stamped addressed envelope if you write to me:

Hazel Chesterman-Phillips
42 Flower Lane
Mill Hill
London
NW7 2JL

BIBLIOGRAPHY

Amelar *First Book on Male Infertility*. Available from Anthony Hirsh FRCS, 55 Wimpole Street, London, W1.

Bathakur, I. K. *A Natural Approach towards the Predetermination of Sex*. Shillong, 1976.

Bennet, N. *Sex Selection of Children*. Academic Press, 1983.

Billings, F. and J. *The Learner's Guide to the Billings Method*. (NAOMI), National Association of Ovulation Instructors, 1984.

Commission for Racial Equality *The Sorrow in my Heart*. College Hill Press, 1993.

Cooper, W. *The Fertile Years*. Hutchinson (Arrow), 1978.

Darwin, C. *Notebooks*. OU Course A 381, OU Press, 1981.

Davies, S. 'Sex of One . . .' *The Guardian*, 19.4.88.

Giesel, J. 'Population.' *Encyclopaedia Americana*, 1984.

Hardy, T. *Jude the Obscure*. Macmillan, 1986.

Health Education Authority *Smoking and Pregnancy*. Health Education Authority, 1993.

Hewitt, J. *Diet Papers*. 1994.

Human Fertilisation and Embryology Authority Consultation Document, 1993.

Inglis, J. K. *A Text Book of Human Biology*. Pergamon Press, 1976.

Kennedy, P. *Preparing for the Twenty-first Century*. HarperCollins, 1993.

Kuhn, T. *The Structure of Scientific Revolutions*, University of Chicago Press, 1970.

Leonard, W. E. *Empedocles: Fragments in Greek and English*. Chicago Open Court Publishing Co., 1908.

Malthus, T. *Essay on the Principle of Population as it effects the Future Improvements of Society*, 1798. Macmillan, 1990.

Miller, S. K. 'Warning: smoking may damage your sperm.' *New Scientist*, 17.10.92.

Open University *Science Foundation Course, Units 16–20*. OU Press, 1970.

Papa, F. and L. F. *Boy or Girl? Choosing your Child through Diet*, Souvenir Press, 1984.

Phillips, H. *Girl or Boy? I Chose my Child*. Chesterman, 1980.

Phillips, H. with Tessa H. *Girl or Boy? Your Chance to Choose*. Thorsons/Harper Collins, 1995.

Popper, K. *The Logic of Scientific Discovery*. Hutchinson, 1959.

Population Concern Annual Report, 1994.

Porter, E. H. *Pollyanna*, 1913.

Roberts, J. *Mastering Human Biology*. Macmillan, 1991.

Rose, S. *The Chemistry of Life*. Penguin, 1970.

Royal College of Physicians *The Medical Consequences of Alcohol Abuse*. Tavistock Publications, 1987.

Shettles, I. B. with David Rorvik. *Your Baby's Sex. Now You Can Choose*. Donald Mead, USA 1970, UK 1980.

Stoppard, M. *Pregnancy and Birth Book*. Dorling Kindersley, 1991.

Warnock, M. *The Report of Commission of Enquiry into Human Fertilization*. DHSS. 1980.

Wingate, P. *Medical Encyclopaedia*. Penguin, 1978.

Winston, R. *Getting Pregnant*. Anaya Publishers, 1989.

PUBLISHER'S CREDITS

Extract from 'The "y" factor in male sperm' by Saffron Davies reproduced by permission of the *Guardian*.

Extract from the *Encyclopedia Americana*, 1985 Edition. Copyright 1985 by Grolier Incorporated. Reprinted by permission.

Extract from *Preparing for the Twenty-first Century* by Paul Kennedy and published by HarperCollins reproduced by permission of David Higham Associates.

INDEX